EDUCATIONAL OUTCOMES:
ASSESSMENT OF QUALITY—
AN ANNOTATED BIBLIOGRAPHY

Pub. No. 18-2189

National League for Nursing • New York

Developed in conjunction with the
accreditation outcomes project
funded by the Helene Fuld Health Trust

ISBN 0-88737-372-0

Manufactured in the United States of America

CONTENTS

PROJECT STAFF

Project Director: Carolyn F. Waltz, PhD, RN, FAAN
Professor and Coordinator for Evaluation
School of Nursing
The University of Maryland
Baltimore, Maryland

Project Manager: Sylvia E. Hart, PhD, RN
Dean
College of Nursing
The University of Tennessee, Knoxville
Interim Director
Division of Education and
Accreditation Services
National League for Nursing
New York, New York

Research Team: Carl Miller, DNSc, RN
Professor
School of Nursing
University of Alabama at Birmingham

Rebecca Dean, MS, RN
Doctoral Student
School of Nursing
University of Maryland
Baltimore, Maryland

Harriet Moore, MS, RN
Doctoral Student
School of Nursing
University of Maryland
Baltimore, Maryland

Lois Neuman, MS, RN
Doctoral Candidate
College of Education
University of Maryland
College Park, Maryland

Barbara Sylvia, MS, RN
Doctoral Candidate
School of Nursing
University of Maryland
Baltimore, Maryland

FOREWORD

Assessment of educational outcomes and accountability for the quality of the products of educational programs are interrelated concepts that have become increasingly important in recent years. Questions about the quality and relevance of educational programs are being asked at every level, from preschool to postdoctoral, by a variety of publics and constituencies. While it is true that quality issues at one level should never be considered less important than those occurring at any other level, accountability for quality does have a particular and unique importance in postsecondary education; with a few notable exceptions, it is at this level that society's leaders are prepared.

It is clearly reasonable to hold accountable for quality and relevance those associated with the general or liberalizing experiences of higher education. It is, however, imperative that those responsible for programs that prepare practicing professionals are able to assess, measure, and report to interested individuals and groups the extent to which their programs are preparing safe, competent, well educated, and appropriately skilled practitioners.

Nursing is, after all, a career in the mainstream of the health care delivery system. It is therefore incumbent upon those associated with and responsible for the preparation of nurses that program quality be systematically monitored, measured, and documented.

The annotated bibliography presented on the pages that follow is a compilation of research projects, journal articles, measurement instruments, and other information about what has occurred or is occurring relative to assessing student educational outcomes in general and nursing education outcomes in particular. The bibliography is the first of several products that will emerge from The Helene Fuld Health Trust Accreditation Outcomes Project which is being implemented by the National League for Nursing. The bibliography should be a helpful resource as nurse educators respond to the challenge of accountability that is inherent in their roles.

Sylvia E. Hart, PhD, RN
Project Manager

PREFACE

The Helene Fuld Health Trust is the world's largest charitable fund devoted exclusively to the welfare of student nurses. Marine Midland Bank, N.A., acting as Trustee of the Helene Fuld Health Trust since 1969, has awarded more than $33 million in grants. The Trust has supported student nurses by providing financial assistance to a broad range of nursing education programs and projects at more than two hundred individual nursing schools throughout the United States and overseas. While this kind of support to schools and programs will continue, the Trust is now expanding its focus to include projects that are national in scope, thereby benefitting all nursing programs.

The Accreditation Outcomes Project is the first of such national projects. The Trust, by funding this project that is being conducted by the National League for Nursing, has made visible its commitment to the enhancement of quality in nursing education programs at every level and location. The Project represents an effort to respond to the concerns and recommendations about quality in higher education that are included in the Carnegie Report entitled, "A Nation Prepared: Teachers for the 21st Century," and other recent publications dealing with the status of higher education in America. It is expected that the findings and recommendations resulting from the Accreditation Outcomes Project will be incorporated into nursing education. The result will be improved nursing care and the patient will be the ultimate beneficiary.

The following annotated bibliography, which is part of the Accreditation Outcomes Project, includes readily available articles on the current state of the art in assessing student outcomes of professional education programs in general and nursing education programs in particular. The articles are pertinent to associate, baccalaureate, diploma, or master's degree nursing education programs and are available through journals, projects, and unpublished research reports accessed through computer data bases such as Educational Resources Information Center(ERIC).

Alan S. Trench
Chairman of the Helene Fuld
   Health Trust
Vice President
Marine Midland Bank, N.A.

OVERVIEW OF THE ACCREDITATION OUTCOMES PROJECT

Nurses have begun to give serious attention to the need to document the outcomes of educational programs in a way that will appropriately reflect variations in the quality and/or effectiveness of programs and services across education and practice settings. The student is the major outcome of the educational process. Hence, the results of reliable and valid measures of students' knowledge, attitudes, and performances upon completion of an educational program, especially in a practice based profession such as nursing, are essential if decisions regarding the programs' quality and effectiveness are to be tenable.

While attention has focused on the need for the measurement of nursing student outcomes, actual efforts in this regard for the most part have been quite limited and narrow in view. Recognizing the need for more work in this area, the Helene Fuld Health Trust, an organization committed to supporting projects that will contribute to the education of student nurses, awarded funds to the National League for Nursing to conduct the Accreditation Outcomes Project. The project consists of a two-year study designed to identify and examine student outcome data as a quality measure. The ultimate goal of the project is to provide those who establish nursing program accreditation criteria—that is, persons with accredited nursing programs—with the information necessary to expand the focus of these accreditation criteria from antecedents and processes to include outcomes. More specifically, the study is designed to identify and define desired student outcomes and to include assessment of these outcomes in the accreditation process without neglecting the assessment of such quantitative student outcomes as test scores and grade point averages.

In order to facilitate the most salient positive impact on the profession of nursing, project efforts are directed toward production of the following:

1. A series of publications presenting the 'state of the art' of the measurement of student outcomes in nursing education. These publications will reflect results from three study activities: (1) the critical review of published and unpublished literature regarding the measurement of student outcomes in nursing and other fields; (2) a survey of all diploma, associate, baccalaureate, and masters' degree programs in nursing; and (3) a content analysis of a representative sample of schools' accreditation self studies. These activities were designed to ascertain information regarding which student outcomes are currently being assessed, the tools and other

methods being employed to assess student outcomes, how results are being used to make decisions regarding the quality and effectiveness of the nursing education program, and the student outcomes nursing administrators and faculty believe ought to be assessed. Implications for documenting the outcomes of nursing education within the context of accreditation will be identified, the relevance of student outcome measurement to accreditation and program quality will be established, and guidelines and recommendations for criteria development will be generated.

2. A directory indexing individual activities for documenting student outcomes. The directory will include the variables being measured, the names and locations of the programs where these variables are being measured, and the name of a contact person. The directory will serve as a mechanism for developing networking among schools.

3. The annotated bibliography contained herein presents literature sources for information regarding educational outcome measurement in general and in nursing and other selected fields.

4. A compendium of tools and methods for documenting nursing education outcomes.

5. A prototype for assessing or measuring student outcome variables including specific steps for determining the reliability and validity of instruments or tools designed to measure cognitive, affective, and performance variables.

The results of this study will assist the National League for Nursing and other accrediting bodies to assess a full array of student outcomes in addition to examining the educational process. Study findings will be useful in (1) translating schools' missions and needs-assessment data into specific goals, objectives, and measurable student outcomes; (2) developing procedures to measure schools' success in achieving goals and desired student outcomes; (3) providing a standard method for collecting, organizing, and analyzing accreditation data in student outcome data files; and (4) introducing procedures for using the student outcome data for continuing education, policy making, strategic planning, and resource allocation.

Study data will also serve faculty in higher education who are responsible for quality assurance, as a guide to tailoring programs for diverse student populations, and as a guide for instituting more goal-directed, management-by-objective strategies that have applications in a wide variety of programs.

Carolyn F. Waltz, PhD, RN
Project Director

1 ACADEMIC ACHIEVEMENT

Grades, Grade Point Average

Aldag, J., & Rose, S. (1983). Relationship of age, American College Testing scores, grade point average and state board examination scores. *Research in Nursing and Health, 6*, 69–73.

> Study examined the relationship between age and American College Testing (ACT) scores to college grade point average and state board examination scores for 787 persons admitted to an associate degree program over a ten-year period.

Bell, J. G., Simons, S. A., & Norris, J. (1983). An alternative pathway to BSN. *Nurse Educator, 8*(4), 34–38.

> Article describes a non-traditional BSN program—an intensive 44-week curriculum that prepares graduates for clinical or postgraduate work in nursing. The program was designed to facilitate career change into nursing for people who already have a bachelor's degree in an area other than nursing. Non-traditional graduates performed as well as traditional graduates and were socialized equally well into the professional role.

Burgess, G. (1980). The self-concept of undergraduate nursing students in relation to clinical performance and selected biographical variables. *Journal of Nursing Education, 19*(3), 37–44.

> Undergraduate nursing students completed the Tennessee Self-Concept Scale in order to test the possibility of a relationship between self-concept and clinical performance, attrition, and selected biographical factors.

Edmondson, M. A. E. (1977). The relationship between self-concept and achievement in nursing education. *Dissertation Abstract International*, 37, 1178-B. (University Microfilms No. 76-21, 455).

> This study sought to determine the relationship between self-concept, as measured by the Tennessee Self-Concept Scale, and academic achievement as measured by clinical grade, theory grade, and standardized achievement test scores.

1

Hayes, E. R. (1981). Prediction of academic success in baccalaureate nursing education programs. *Journal of Nursing Education, 20*(6), 4–8.

> The purpose of the study was to determine the validity of selected cognitive variables to the additive value of certain uncognitive variables in predicting academic success as measured by completion of the BSN program.
> Findings suggest cognitive variables are the most powerful predictors of academic success. Tools used to measure non-cognitive variables were the California Psychological Inventory (CPI) and the Survey of Interpersonal Values (SIV).
> CPI assesses: dominance, capacity for status, sociability, social presence, self-acceptance, sense of well-being, responsibility, self-control, tolerance, good impression, psychological-mindedness, flexibility, and femininity.
> SIV assesses: areas of support, conformity, recognition, benevolence, and leadership.

Higgs, Z. R. (1984). Predicting success in nursing: From prototype to pragmatics. *Western Journal of Nursing Research, 6*, 77–95.

> Study to determine the degree admission criteria individually and in combination predict success in generic baccalaureate programs using samples of 1974, 1975, and 1976 entering classes and the merged data from the three classes (N = 507). Indicators of success included program completion; grade point average for nursing courses; grade point averages for pathophysiology and pharmacology courses; and clinical course grade point average as reflected by written examinations, papers, and projects.

Hilbert, G., & Allen, L. R. (1985). The effect of social support on educational outcomes. *Journal of Nursing Education, 24*(2), 48–52.

> This study examined the relationship among social support, test anxiety, self-esteem, and the educational outcomes of grade point averages and NCLEX-RN scores.

Jones, F. C. (1977). A comparative study in self-concept of Jackson Community College students who remained to completion, April, 1974 versus those who withdrew before completion, Fall, 1973. *Dissertation Abstracts International*, 38, 2509A (University Microfilms No. 77-23, 987).

> The Tennessee Self-Concept Scale was used to compare the differences between the mean scores of students who withdrew and those who graduated.

Kramer, G. A., & DeMarais, D. R. (1986). Trends in academic qualifications and performance of dental students. *Journal of Dental Education, 50*, 213–220.

> This study examined the academic qualifications and dental school performance measures of students enrolled at public and private dental schools during the five-year period beginning in 1980.

Moser, R. S. (1984). Perceived role taking behavior and course grades in junior year college nursing students. *Journal of Nursing Education, 23*(7), 294–297.

> Junior nursing students volunteered to complete the Peer Role Taking Questionnaire. A role taking score was computed for each subject and compared to the individual's grade point average.

Munro, B. H., & Krauss, J. B. (1985). The success of non-BSNs in graduate nursing programs. *Journal of Nursing Education, 24*, 192–196.

> An ex post facto study to determine any difference in success among the three groups of individuals admitted to the two-year master's program at Yale. Non-nurse college graduates, BSNs, and nurses with a non-nursing baccalaureate degree were compared on their theoretical and clinical grades at the end of the first- and second-year specialty programs.

Oliver, D. H. (1985). The relationship of selected admission criteria to the academic success of associate degree nursing students. *Journal of Nursing Education, 24*, 197–206.

> An ex post facto study to determine which of 11 independent variables most effectively predicted academic success, as measured by first-quarter grade point average and successful or nonsuccessful program completion; and to determine if there were clusters of independent variables that better predicted first-quarter grade point average and program completion than did single independent variables for 141 students of one ADN program.

Paolillo, J. G. (1982). The predicted validity of selected admissions variables relative to grade point average earned in a master's of business administration program. *Educational and Psychological Measurement, 42*, 1163–1167.

> Brief review of research using stepwise linear regression analysis to identify variables that explain significant amounts of variance in graduate grade point average for 220 graduates of one program.

Sime, M. A., Corcoran, S. A., & Libera, M. (1983). BSN vs. non-BSN students and success in graduate study. *Journal of Nursing Education, 22,* 190–194.

> Study of the entry and progression characteristics of graduate students (nurses) with baccalaureate degrees in fields other than nursing (non-BSN) as compared to characteristics of students whose baccalaureate degrees were in nursing (BSN). Progression characteristics included cumulative and final grade point averages and faculty evaluations of students' abilities.

Smith, A. W., & Allen, W. R. (1984). Modeling black student academic performance in higher education. *Research in Higher Education, 21,* 210–225.

> The National Study for Black College Students (NSBCS) was employed to develop a model that distinguishes between high and low performing black undergraduates attending four-year institutions. In the NSBCS sample (N = 695) discriminant function analysis identified several institutional and student characteristics which were related to black students' educational outcomes of self reported and grade point averages and self reported occupational aspirations.

Suiddick, D. E., & Collins, B. A. (1982). A validation of the use of American College Testing, proficiency examination program for advanced upper-division placement of nursing students graduated from hospital-based (diploma) nursing programs. *Educational and Psychological Measurement, 42,* 1177–1179.

> Brief summary of comparison of cumulative grade point average of 76 ADN graduates and 21 diploma graduates who had entered an upper-division program for BSNs in the fall of 1979. Diploma graduates were required to pass three ACT Proficiency Examination Program tests whereas ADN graduates were not required to take the tests.

Zagar, R., Arbit, J., & Wengel, W. (1982). Personality factors as predictors of grade point average and graduation from nursing school. *Educational and Psychological Measurement, 42,* 1169–1175.

> A brief review of research to determine the predictive validity of the Edwards Personal Preference Schedule and the Minnesota Multiphasic Personality Inventory relative to that afforded by the American College Testing Program Assessment composite score in forecasting success in a three-year hospital-based nursing program as measured by grade point average.

Standardized Tests

Nursing

Breyer, J. (1984). The comprehensive nursing achievement test as a predictor of performance on the NCLEX-RN. *Nursing and Health Care, 5,* 193–195.

> Study to assess the ability of the 1982 edition of the Comprehensive Nursing Achievement Test to predict scores on the NCLEX-RN. Presents equations that could predict NCLEX-RN scores from the clinical content advisory subscores reported in the 1983 edition of the Comprehensive Nursing Achievement Test.

Dell, M. A., & Halpin, G. (1984). Predictors of success in nursing school and on state board examinations in a predominately black baccalaureate nursing program. *Journal of Nursing Education, 23,* 147–150.

> Relationships between Scholastic Aptitude Test scores, high school grade point average, National League for Nursing Pre-Nursing Examination scores, college grade point average, and state board examination scores were examined using discriminant analysis procedures.

Larkin, P. G. (1977). *Admission test results as criteria for entrance into the nursing program and regression analysis of entrance tests as predictors of success in nursing.* Largo, MD: Prince George's Community College. (ERIC Document Reproduction Service No. ED 143 338).

> Twenty-two-page research report on an analysis of the records of 159 nursing graduates of 1976 on demographic variables, state board examination subtest scores, Comparative Guidance and Placement tests (CGP) taken at entry, process variables, grade point average, and nursing and science course repeats. Analysis was for the purpose of establishing a more equitable admissions selection process that could lead to successful completion of the five-part state board examination.

Quick, M. M., Krupa, K. C., & Whitley, T. W. (1985). Using admission data to predict success on the NCLEX-RN in a baccalaureate program. *Journal of Professional Nursing, 1,* 364–368.

> Study in which graduates of a baccalaureate program were divided into two groups on the basis of whether they passed or failed the NCLEX-RN. Using discriminant analysis of grade point average at the end of the freshman year, scores on the verbal portion of the Scholastic Aptitude Test and

grades in an anatomy and physiology course were directly related to the NCLEX-RN performance; general chemistry and biochemistry grades were inversely related.

Sharp, T. G. (1984). An analysis of the relationship of seven selected variables to state board test pool examination performance of the University of Tennessee, Knoxville, College of Nursing. *Journal of Nursing Education, 23,* 57–63.

> An analysis of seven variables (high school grade point average; college of nursing grade point average; and American College Test assessment standard scores for English, Mathematics, Social Studies, and Composite) to pass/fail on the state board test pool examination (SBTPE) and to the five SBTPE subexam scores for 572 graduates of one BSN program.

Stankovich, M. J. (1977). *The statistical predictability of academic performance of registered nursing student at Macomb.* Warren, MI: Macomb County Community College. (ERIC Document Reproduction Service No. ED 161 501).

> Forty-three page report of a study to determine (1) whether there was a significant relationship between grades earned in individual nursing courses and the scores earned on corresponding subsets of the state board examination for nursing graduates and (2) whether a student's success could be predicted from admission characteristics. Linear relationships were computed using a sample of students/graduates (N = 130) of one program.

St. Thomas, S. (1982). *An analysis of the relationship between the first semester grade point average and the state board nursing scores of Vermont College graduates.* Nova University. (ERIC Document Reproduction Service No. ED 214 572).

> A study to analyze the relationship of the first semester grade point average (GPA) and scores on the state board examination.

Washburn, G. (1980). *Relationship of achievement test scores and state board performance in a diploma nursing program.* Indiana University at South Bend (ERIC Document Reproduction Service No. ED 203 752).

> The relationship between National League for Nursing (NLN) achievement test scores and performance on the state board test pool examination (SBTPE) was studied with 165 graduates of a diploma nursing program between 1976 and 1978. Results indicated NLN achievement test scores had a highly significant correlation with SBTPE results.

Whitley, M. P., & Chadwick, P. L. (1986). Baccalaureate education and NCLEX: The causes of success. *Journal of Nursing Education, 25,* 94–101.

> Research study to investigate causal and correlational relationships between scores on the NCLEX and conceptual and experimental areas of the curriculum, student potential, and student performance for 176 BSN graduates of one program.

Wisenbaker, S., & Lee, M. (1986). Predicting success. *AD Nurse, 1*(5), 15–17.

> A study to determine if a significant relationship existed between nursing students' scores on the Mosby Assess Test and the students' scores on the National Council Licensure Examination (NCLEX-RN). Bivariate correlation using Pearson product moment correlation revealed a significant positive correlation (r = .67). The sample consisted of 172 AD nursing students of one program.

Woodham, R., & Taube, K. (1986). Relationship of nursing program predictors and success on the NCLEX-RN examination for licensure in a selected associate degree program. *Journal of Nursing Education, 25,* 112–117.

> An ex post facto correlational study to determine the relationship of selected admission criteria and performance in the integrated nursing major didactic courses of associate science in nursing degree programs as predictors for performance on the licensing examination for registered nurses.

Yocom, C. J., & Scherubel, J. C. (1985). Selected pre-admission and academic correlates of success on state board examinations. *Journal of Nursing Education, 24,* 244–249.

> A retrospective study to examine students' performances prior to and following admission to a baccalaureate nursing program in comparison with their performance on the individual sections of the state board test pool examinations (SBE) and an overall assessment of pass–fail on the SBE for 139 class of 1980 graduates of one program.

Non-Nursing

Farquhar, L. J., Haf, J., & Kotabe, K. (1986). Effect of two pre-clinical curricula on NBME Part I Examination performance. *Journal of Medical Education, 61,* 368–373.

> Comparison of the effects of two teaching methodologies (lecture versus problem based) on the student's performance on the National Board of

Medical Examiners Part 1 Examination which is a graduation requirement at Michigan State University College of Human Medicine.

Kitabchi, G. (1985, March/April). *Multivariate analysis of urban community college student performance on the ACT College Outcomes Measurement Program Test.* Paper presented at the Annual Meeting of the American Educational Research Association, Chicago, IL. (ERIC Document Reproduction Service No. ED 261 091).

 Fifteen-page report of a study that examined the relationship and relative importance of selected variables to successful performance of 696 urban college students of one college on the ACT College Outcomes Measures Program Test (ACT COMP). With the exception of nursing and allied health (programs with selective admission criteria), older students, white ethnic groups and transfer degree students had higher ACT COMP performance than their counterparts.

Larson, D. B., Orleans, C. S., & Houpt, J. L. (1980). Evaluating a clinical psychiatry course using process and outcome measures. *Journal of Medical Education, 55,* 1006–1012.

 Objectives of the study were to describe actual clinical clerkship activities and a variety of learning outcomes overall and across rotations. Four variables of learning outcomes were measured: knowledge, perceived skill, attitude, and student satisfaction. An evaluation was done of overall outcomes, a comparison of outcomes across rotations, and an examination of relationships between different types of outcomes.

Rinchuse, D. J., & Zullo, T. (1986). The cognitive level demands of a dental school's predoctoral didactic examinations. *Journal of Dental Education, 50,* 167–171.

 A sample of the test items was selected from the entire population of predoctoral written examination questions administered by the University of Pittsburgh, School of Dental Medicine. The sample test items were classified according to Bloom's taxonomy of educational objectives. Research questions examined (1) the number and percentage of test items represented by each of the six major levels of Bloom's taxonomy of educational objectives of the cognitive domain; (2) whether there was a difference in the student cognitive level demands between basic science subject test items and clinical subject test items; and (3) whether there was a difference in the student cognitive level demands among freshman, sophomore, and junior year test items.

Program Completion

Donsky, A. P., & Judge, A. J. (1981, May). *Academic and nonacademic characteristics as predictors of persistance in an associate degree program.* Paper presented at the Annual Forum of the Association for Institutional Research, Minneapolis, MN. (ERIC Document Reproduction Service No. ED 205 076).

> Academic variables (American College Testing Program standard scores, National League for Nursing rank scores, high school and previous college grade averages) and nonacademic variables (marital status, sex, admission pattern, age, prior nursing type experience, study habits, attitudes, and interests) were used to predict persistence in the nursing program at Lakeland Community College, Ohio.

Jacobs, A. M., Young, D. M., & dela Cruz, F. A. (1985, June). *An evaluation model for prototype nursing continuing education models.* Paper presented at the Measurement of Clinical and Nursing Outcomes Conference, New Orleans, LA.

> Using a basic input, process, and outcomes model, the author suggests a method for measuring the effectiveness of continuing education programs. Suggested outcome variables are total number of students who complete the program, drop-outs, and self-reports of program satisfaction and learning application. Also used are a criterion-referenced knowledge test and performance rating.

Roediger, J. L. (1983). Relationship of self-concept, life change stress, and student attrition in community nursing programs. *Dissertation Abstracts International, 43,* 3825-A. (University Microfilms No. DA 8308640).

> This study examined the relationship of self-concept, life change, stress, and student attrition in community college practical nursing and associate degree nursing programs.

Tripp, A., & Duffey, M. (1981). Discriminant analysis to predict graduation–nongraduation in a master's degree program in nursing. *Research in Nursing and Health, 4,* 345–353.

> Discriminant analysis was used to predict graduation and two categories of nongraduation from readily available admissions data of a nursing master's degree program. Predictors included baccalaureate grade point average and Graduate Record Examination verbal and quantitative scores. Criterion categories were composed of 102 graduates, 103 individuals who dropped out of the program, and 65 individuals who were not accepted into the program.

Weinstein, E. L. (1980). Characteristics of the successful nursing student. *Journal of Nursing Education, 19*(3), 53–59.

> A study to investigate demographic variables, behavioral antecedents, and selection criteria most characteristic of the successful nursing student. Success is defined as passing the first year of a two-year diploma nursing program in Canada.

2 CLINICAL PERFORMANCE

Nursing Students

Bondy, K. N. (1984). Clinical evaluation of student performance: The effects of criteria on accuracy and reliability. *Research in Nursing and Health, 7,* 25–33.

> The purpose of this study was to determine whether faculty (experienced and inexperienced) who had specific criteria for each point of a five-point scale would more accurately evaluate a videotaped student performance than faculty (experienced and inexperienced) who used the five-point scale without criteria.

Cronin-Stubbs, D., & Mathews, J. G. (1982). A clinical performance evaluation tool for a process-oriented nursing curriculum. *Nurse Educator, 7*(4), 24–29.

> This article discussed the process of developing and implementing a formative and summative clinical evaluation tool to assess undergraduate students' ability to use the nursing process in a variety of health care settings.

Field, W. E., Gallman, L., Nicholson, R., & Dreker, M. (1984). Clinical competencies of baccalaureate students. *Journal of Nursing Education, 23,* 284–293.

> Sixty-four NLN-accredited baccalaureate programs responded to a request for all of the clinical objectives used in their programs. The objectives were sorted into three domains (cognitive, affective, psychomotor) and compared and contrasted.

Lee, H. A., & Strong, K. A. (1985). Using nursing diagnosis to describe the clinical competence of baccalaureate and associate degree graduating students: A comparative study. *Image: The Journal of Nursing Scholarship, 17*(3), 82–85.

> This study used a nursing diagnosis framework to examine perceived clinical competence of students graduating with associate degrees and those graduating with baccalaureate degrees and to compare the students' perceptions of competence with the expectations of their faculty members.

11

McBride, H., Littlefield, J., & Garman, R. E. (1981). A simulation method measuring psychomotor skills. *Evaluation and the Health Profession, 4*, 295–305.

> Describes the development and use of a simulation method to assess proficiency in performing 18 psychomotor nursing skills in one undergraduate baccalaureate nursing program. Criterion-referenced checklists were developed and dependability coefficients based upon generalizability theory are reported.

McCloskey, J. C. (1981). The effects of nursing education on job effectiveness: An overview of the literature. *Research in Nursing and Health, 4*, 355–373.

> An overview of the published studies on the effectiveness of nursing education as it relates to job performance. Selected literature is reviewed and divided into three areas of study: competency, performance, and quality of care. Suggestions for research direction and improvements are discussed. A comprehensive bibliography is included.

McMillan, S. C. (1985). A comparison of professional performance examination scores of graduating associate and baccalaureate degree nursing students. *Research in Nursing and Health, 8*, 167–172.

> The Professional Performance Examination of the New York Regents External Degrees in Nursing Program was administered to graduating seniors from associate and baccalaureate degree programs in order to compare the graduates on leadership, collaboration, research, and management of client care.

Palermo, M., & Sokoloff, J. (1979). *Final report of development of a clinical performance tool.* Sewell, NJ: Gloucester Community College. (ERIC Document Reproduction Service No. ED 187 846).

> Seventy-three-page report of a research project to develop a criterion-referenced test of clinical nursing performance that could evaluate skill mastery; to establish the degree of interrater agreement; to establish congruent validity; and to develop manuals for students' and evaluators' use. The report contains numerous tables and a listing of the critical requirements for basic nursing skills.

Reynolds, W., & Cormack, D. (1982). Clinical teaching: An evaluation of a problem-oriented approach to psychiatric nurse education. *Journal of Advanced Nursing, 7*, 231–237.

> This article describes the use of a problem-oriented approach to the evaluation of students in a psychiatric setting. It did not employ any comparisons or research methods in the evaluations.

Squier, R. W. (1981). The reliability and validity of rating scales in assessing the clinical progress of psychiatric nursing students. *International Journal of Nursing Studies, 18*(3), 157–169.

> The purposes of this study were to (1) develop a reliable scale for assessing student nurses' clinical progress during a three-year program in a psychiatric hospital; (2) evaluate the validity of assessments of clinical progress by comparing them with state final written and practical exams; and (3) determine the relationship between final ratings and certain demographic data.

Whelan, E. (1982). Increasing clinical proficiency: A summer clinical course. *Nurse Educator, 7*(5), 28–31.

> The author describes the development, implementation, and evaluation of a clinical minicourse. Evaluation of the course was based on a clinical performance tool and student self-evaluation.

Nursing Graduates

Bolin, S. E., & Hogle, E. L. (1984). Relationship between college success and employer competency ratings for graduates of a baccalaureate nursing program. *Journal of Nursing Education, 23*, 15–20.

> An ex post facto correlational study to examine the relationship between preentrance test scores, clinical experience grades, grade point averages, and state board test pool examination scores to competency ratings of graduates by their employers one year after graduation. The study uses a faculty-constructed questionnaire containing 12 nursing abilities to be rated on a five-point scale.

Boronies, D, I., & Neuman, N. A. (1981). Graduate nurse transition program. *American Journal of Nursing, 81*(10), 1832–1835.

> This article described the development, implementation, and evaluation of a program to assist new graduates in their transition to staff nurse. Evaluation forms were designed by the authors.

DeBack, V., & Mentkowski, M. (1986). Does the baccalaureate make a difference?: Differentiating nurse performance by education and experience. *Journal of Nursing Education, 25*, 275–285.

> Study to test the hypotheses that (1) baccalaureate nurse graduates perform more nursing competencies than associate degree or diploma nurses and (2) nurses with more nursing experience perform more nursing com-

petencies. The competencies were conceptualizing, ego stamina, ego strength, independence, influencing, teaching, reflective thinking, positive expectations, and helping. Analysis of data collected from 83 nurses using a peer nomination questionnaire, a job element inventory, a biographical questionnaire, and the McClelland Behavioral Event Interview indicated significant differences in several competencies based on a level of education and experience.

Goodwin, L., Prescott, P., Jacox, A., & Collar, M. (1981). The nurse practitioner rating form, part II, methodological development. *Nurse Research, 30*(5), 270–276.

This series of studies was conducted to establish the reliability and validity of the Nurse Practitioner Rating Form (NPRF) in various settings and circumstances.

Gullickson, B. (1985). *Development of a simulated clinical performance examination.* Paper presented at the Measurement of Clinical and Nursing Outcome Conference, New Orleans, LA.

Using a checklist for direct observation and chart audit, this paper traced the development of a criterion-referenced measure for assessing clinical performance as an outcome of nursing education.

Hegedus, K. S., Balasco, E. M., & Black, A. S. (1985). *Examination of clinical performance.* Paper presented at the Measurement of Clinical and Nursing Outcomes Conference, New Orleans, LA.

This was a report of the development of a criterion-referenced measure used to assess clinical performance among professional nurses. Using clinical practice, clinical leadership, professional growth, continuing education, and involvement in nursing research as indicators, the measure encompassed both subject self-report and judgement of the immediate nurse manager for assessing clinical performance outcomes.

Holzemer, W. L., Schleutermann, J. A., Farrand, L. L., & Miller, A. G. (1981). Simulations as a measure of nurse practitioners' problem-solving skills. *Nursing Research, 30*(3), 139–144.

A national sample of 79 family and adult nurse practitioners completed 6 instruments designed to validate clinical simulation of patient management problems.

Ignatavicius, D. (1983). Clinical competence of new graduates: A study to measure performance. *The Journal of Continuing Education in Nursing, 14*(4), 17–20.

Nineteen graduate nurses were evaluated six months after participating in a transition orientation program at one hospital. A competency index, developed by the investigator, was used to assess the graduate nurses. The graduate nurses and their head nurses both completed the competency index for each subject.

Jones, L. C., Soeken, K. L., & Guberski, T. D. (1986). Development of an instrument to measure self-reported leadership behaviors of nurse practitioners. *Journal of Professional Nursing,* 2(3), 180–185.

> The article reports on the development of the Nurse Practitioner Leadership Questionnaire—a five dimensional instrument constructed to measure self-reported leadership behavior in nurse practitioners. Content validity and item clarity were assessed by five nurse practitioner faculty members. Results from the revised instrument administration are being used to structure the teaching of leadership content in a master's-level nurse practitioner curriculum.

Keiffer, J. S. (1984). Selecting technical skills to teach for competency. *Journal of Nursing Education, 23*(5), 198–203.

> The author surveyed staff nurses in a local hospital to find the skills most used and needed by graduate nurses.

Longsdale, A. J., Dennis, N. C., Hooke, S., & Norvilas, C. (1982). *Evaluating the nursing performance of college and hospital graduates: Procedures outcomes and issues. A report of the Nursing Education Evaluation Project.* Bently Western Australia: Western Australian Institute of Technology. (ERIC Document Reproduction Service No. ED 226 665).

> One hundred sixty-page research report concerned with the development and testing of procedures and instruments for the evaluation of nursing performance with the limited number of Western Australian Institute graduates (N = 9) who entered the workforce in 1981 and with a comparison group of graduates (N = 18) from hospital-based courses. Tests and interview forms included.

McCloskey, J. C. (1983). Nursing education and job effectiveness. *Nursing Research, 32*(1), 53–58.

> Multiple regression study to determine whether nurses with different educational preparation differ in job effectiveness as rated by their head nurses. The sample consisted of 53 practical nurses, 63 associate degree nurses, 134 diploma nurses, and 49 baccalaureate nurses. An educational model of job effectiveness is provided.

McLaughlin, F. E., Carr, J. W., & Delucehi, K. L. (1981). Measurement properties of clinical simulation tests: Hypertension and chronic obstructive pulmonary disease. *Nursing Research, 30*(1), 5–9.

> The reliability and validity of two clinical simulation tests were studied. The same subjects were tested for reliability 60–90 days after the first

testing. Validity was assessed by comparing test scores of two expert panels, comparing test contents with authoritative literature on the diseases and analysis results of test evaluation by all subjects.

Mims, B. C. (1985). *Development of clinical performance examination for critical care nurses.* Paper presented at the Measurement of Clinical and Nursing Outcomes Conference, 1985, New Orleans, LA.

The study looked at the effectiveness of using the Clinical Performance Examination, developed by Morgan and Irby, as a tool for measuring the clinical performance of critical care nurses. The methodology employed was observation by staff development personnel. It was concluded that further refinement of the tool is necessary to increase the value of results.

Nelson, L. F. (1978). Competence of nursing graduates in technical, communicative and administrative skills. *Nursing Research, 27*, 121–124.

The survey examined baccalaureate, diploma, and associate degree nursing program graduates regarding their perceptions of their competence in technical, communicative, and administrative skills and their supervisors' perceptions of the graduates' competency.

Ramsborg, G. C. (1983). Evaluation of clinical performance, Part II. *Journal of American Association of Nurse Anesthetists, 51*(2), 167–174.

The author describes the development, implementation, and evaluation of the clinical performance of nurse anesthetists. No evaluation of the forms was indicated in the article.

Schoen, D. C. (1983). Predictors of success for ADN graduates. *Nursing Leadership, 6*, 104–112.

An analysis of four principal predictor variables to clinical competency of ADN graduates approximately two and one-half years after graduation as determined by supervisor ratings of the ADN graduates in five areas of competency. Instruments to measure competency included areas of work achievement, position competency, communication skills, cooperation, and work success factors.

Schwirian, P. M. (1978). *Prediction of successful nursing performance part I and part II.* Hyattsville, MD: U.S. Department of Health, Education and Welfare.

Two of three phases of a study conducted to (1) assess the state of the art on the prediction of nursing clinical performance and (2) obtain information from nursing education programs about prediction criteria in use by them. Report contains 22 tables summarizing the 398 studies reviewed.

Schwirian, P. M. (1978). *Prediction of successful nursing performance part III and part IV.* Hyattsville, MD: U.S. Department of Health, Education and Welfare.

> Final phases of a study to ascertain the relative success of a sample of 1975 graduates as ascertained in a self-appraisal and performance appraisal provided by the graduates' immediate supervisors. Numerous tables are included.

Schwirian, P. M. (1978). Evaluating the performance of nurses: A multidimensional approach. *Nursing Research, 27,* 347–351.

> Article describes the development—including content, structure, validity, and reliability—of the Six-Dimensional Scale of Nursing Performance, which consists of a series of 52 behaviors grouped into six performance subscales: leadership, critical care, teaching/collaboration, planning/evaluation, interpersonal relations/communications, and professional development.

Stokes, S. A., Werlin, E. L., Rauckhorst, L., & Gother, A. M. (1981). The development of an evaluation process for technical level competency. *Nursing and Health Care, 2*(4), 192–195, 230.

> Technical level competencies of AD graduates were evaluated by showing the subjects seven videotaped vignettes representing content from the areas of fundamentals, maternal/child, psychiatric, and adult nursing. Multiple choice questions were administered on each vignette.

Sweeney, M. A., & Regan, P. A. (1982). Educators, employees, and new graduates define essential skills for baccalaureate graduates. *The Journal of Nursing Administration, 12*(9), 36–42.

> A list of 291 psychomotor skills was given to subjects in nursing education and nursing service and recent baccalaureate graduates. Using a Q-sort technique, the subjects were asked to categorize the skills into four groups: essential, bonus, graduate, and non-nursing.

Non-nursing Students

Abrahamson, S. (1985). Assessment of student clinical performance. *Evaluation and The Health Profession, 8,* 413–427.

> The article discusses methods of assessing medical students. It identifies computer applications, simulated patients, and the videotape/videodisc as ways to apply more imaginative assessment procedures.

DaRosa, D. A., Dawson-Saunders, B., & Folse, R. (1985). A comparison of objective and subjective measures of clinical competence. *Evaluation and Program Planning, 8,* 327–330.

> The purpose of the study was to determine whether objective performance measures from a simulated patient practical examination were related to faculty's subjective assessments of surgery medical student performance.

Hunskaar, S., & Seim, S. (1984). The effect of a checklist on medical students' exposures to practical skills. *Medical Education, 18,* 439–442.

> This was a study of the effect of a checklist exploring acquisition of practical skills by medical students during the first clinical course in internal medicine. A group of forty-five students using the checklist was compared with two reference groups taking the class before and after the study groups.

Martin, Y. M., Harris, D. L., & Karg, M. B. (1985). Clinical competence of graduating medical students. *Journal of Medical Education, 60,* 919–934.

> This survey was done to determine clinical skills in which graduating medical students should be competent. This allows for comparison of the clinical expectations of practicing physicians and of medical schools regarding medical students.

Petzel, R. A., Harris, I. B., & Masler, D. S. (1982). The empirical validation of clinical teaching strategies. *Evaluation and the Health Professions, 5,* 499–508.

> The purpose of the study was to empirically validate the effectiveness of certain teaching strategies in one introductory medical course by observation and rating of students' clinical performance in areas of communication, history-taking, and physical examination skills at the beginning of subsequent medical course for second-year medical students.

Seefelft, M., & Blumberg, P. (1984). Rating dental students, a comparison of faculty and patient perspectives. *Evaluation and the Health Professions, 7,* 365–374.

> The study compares supervisor and patient perceptions of dental students' clinical performance in areas of interpersonal skills, empathetic behavior, efficiency, ability to inspire confidence, credibility, knowledge base, and other attributes related to professional performance. Postvisit questionnaires were completed by 52 patients and supervisor instructors of dental students.

Wright, H. J., Stanley, M., & Webster, J. (1983). Assessment of cognitive abilities in clinical medicine. *Medical Education, 17,* 31–38.

> This study tests the hypothesis that eight discrete cognitive abilities necessary to clinical practice can be identified and their achievement reliability assessed by short-answer question papers, a method applicable to a large (N = 222) number of students.

Non-nursing Graduates

Fielding, D. W., & Jang, R. (1981). A continuing pharmacy education program. *Evaluation and the Health Professions, 4*(1), 21–28.

> Study measures the effectiveness of a continuing education program developed to enhance a community pharmacist's ability to respond to requests for nonprescription medication by using trained observers to measure the pharmacist's behavior before and after the program.

Niebuhr, B. R., & Lanier, R. A. (1982). Professional performance of physician's assistants. *Evaluation and the Health Professions, 5*(3), 273–282.

> Study of ratings of physician's assistants (N = 56) and their supervisory physicians for comparative purposes. Both were interviewed using an interview instrument developed to cover the performance of the physician's assistant in the major activities of primary care practice.

Norman, G. R., Neufeld, V. R., Walsh, A., Woodward, C. A., & McConvey, G. A. (1985). Measuring physicians performance by using simulated patients. *Journal of Medical Education, 60,* 925–934.

> This is a study of a new approach to the assessment of physicians' performances in practice using simulated patients. Specific performance criteria were established for seven standardized patients by eight family physicians and two specialists. Sample was two cohorts of family physicians. No differences were found between the criteria-setting and the noncriteria-setting physicians, but large differences were found among the criteria, the physicians' performances as indicated by the patient, and the chart data noted by the physician.

3 EMPATHY/COMMUNICATION

Nursing Students

Gagan, J. M. (1983). Methodological notes on empathy. *Advances in Nursing Science, 5*(2), 65–72.

> This paper discusses various problems in measuring and defining empathy. The most widely used tool in nursing studies is the Barett–Lennard Relationship Inventory (BLRI) Empathy Subscale. The author discusses the BLRI and questions the suitability of the empathy subscale.

Johnson, M. H., & Zone, J. B. (1981). Concentrating on the process of learning while teaching clearly defined communication skills. *Journal of Nursing Education, 20*(3), 3–14.

> The authors designed a learning package for ADN students in the psychiatric rotation. The focus was on communication skills; two assessment tools were developed (The Psychiatric Minimal Objective Tool and the Psychiatric Assessment Tool).

Kunst-Wilson, W., Carpenter, L., Poser, A., Venohr, I., and Kushner, K. (1981). Empathic perceptions of nursing students: Self-reported and actual ability. *Research in Nursing and Health, 4*, 283–293.

> The authors used the Kagan's Affective Sensitivity Scale and the Empathic Ability Self-Report Questionnaire to assess undergraduate and graduate students' empathic skills.

Mynatt, S. (1985). Empathy in faculty and students in different types of nursing preparation programs. *Western Journal of Nursing Research, 7*(3), 333–348.

> The relationships and difference between empathy and other characteristics of students and teachers in four types of nursing programs were examined.

21

Nursing Graduates

Brunt, J. H. (1985). An exploration of the relationship between nurses' empathy and technology. *Nursing Administration Quarterly, 9*(4), 69–78.

> The Hogan Empathy Scale and the Perceived Technology Scale (investigator-designed) were used to test the relationship between technology and empathy in nurses from four specialty areas.

Clay, M. (1984). Development of an empathic interaction skills schedule in a nursing context. *Journal of Advanced Nursing, 9,* 343–350.

> Videotapes of nurse-patient interactions were used to teach and assess empathic interaction skills in the classroom and in the clinical situation. The theoretical approach was based on the Carl Rogers approach to communication.

Dawson, C. (1985). Hypertension, perceived clinician empathy and patient self-disclosure. *Research in Nursing and Health, 8,* 191–198.

> The purpose of this study was to compare two groups of chronically ill patients to a control group of nonchronically ill patients on their perceptions of clinician empathy and the importance and difficulty of self-disclosure to health care providers.

Forrest, D. (1983). Analysis of nurses' verbal communication with patients. *Nursing Papers, 15*(3), 48–56.

> The purposes of this study were twofold: (1) construction of an analysis system to provide for the coding of verbal behaviors of the nurse, which facilitated or blocked patient self-exploration and (2) the use of the system by trained coders to code the verbal behaviors used by nurses in videotaped interactions and a comparison between the amount of facilitating and blocking behaviors employed by the nurses.

Hardin, S. B., & Halaris, A. L. (1983). Nonverbal communication of patients and high and low empathy nurses. *Journal of Psychosocial Nursing and Mental Health Services, 21*(1), 14–20.

> Observations were made of the engaging and defensive nonverbal behaviors of patients and nurses. Comparison of the observation scores were made with the patients' ratings of the nurses on the Barrett–Lennard Relationship Inventory.

Hills, M. D., & Knowles, D. (1983). Nurses' levels of empathy with respect in simulation interactions with patients. *International Journal of Nursing Studies, 20*(2), 83–87.

> Videotaped simulations were presented to nurse volunteers. Responses were scored on the empathy and respect scales developed by Carkhuff.

Iwasew, C., & Olson, J. (1985). A comparison of the communication skills of practicing diploma and baccalaureate staff nurses. *Nursing Papers, 17*(2), 38–47.

> The Behavioral Test of Interpersonal Skills for health professions (BTIS) was used to investigate whether differences in communication skills exist between baccalaureate and diploma nurses.

LaMonica, E. L. (1981). Construct validity of an empathy instrument. *Research in Nursing and Health, 4*, 389–400.

> The Empathy Construct Rating Scale was compared to the Carkhuff Index of Communication, the California Psychological Inventory, the Human-Heartedness Questionnaire, the Chapin Social Insight Test, the Philosophy of Human Nature, the Vocabulary Test, and the Tennessee Self-Concept Scale.

Non-nursing Students

Carney, S., & Mitchell, K. R. (1986). Satisfaction of patients with medical students' clinical skills. *Journal of Medical Education, 61*, 374–379.

> A patient satisfaction—dissatisfaction rating scale was developed to measure patients' perceptions of the attitudes and communication skills of medical students at the University of Newcastle, Australia. Specific student characteristics are included.

Dunning, D. G., & Lange, B. M. (1986). Communication tendencies of senior dental students. *Journal of Dental Education, 50*(3), 172–175.

> Study identifies interpersonal behaviors which can be used as a basis for evaluating dental students' communication skills.

Wolfe, F. M. et al. (1984). Meta-analytic evaluation of an interpersonal skills curriculum for medical students: Synthesizing evidence over successive occasions. *Journal of Counseling Psychology, 31*(2), 253–275.

The results of individual evaluations of four successive classes of medical students' performances in communication and interviewing skills were combined and the effect size was determined. Carkhuff's Standard Indexes of Discrimination and Communication were administered before and after interviewing and communication skills training.

4 LOGICAL PROBLEM SOLVING AND DECISION MAKING

Nursing Students

Griei, M. R., & Schnitzler, C. P. (1979). Nurses propensity to risk. *Nursing Research, 28*(3), 186–191.

> Looking at all levels of nursing education, this study looked at nurses' propensity for risk taking using both number judgement and nursing judgement as indicators. The authors concluded that such propensity depends on education level and the situation at hand. They also indicated that the study had important implications for the processing of information in making patient care decisions.

Jenkins, H. M. (1985). *Clinical decision making measured by the Clinical Decision Making in Nursing Scale.* Paper presented at the Measurement of Clinical and Nursing Outcomes Conference, New Orleans, Louisiana.

> The study looked at clinical decision making based on the results of a summated rating scale employing self-report on four basic criteria: (1) search for options or alternatives; (2) canvassing of objectives and values; (3) evaluation and re-evaluation of consequences; and (4) search for information and unbiased assimilation of new information. Results were somewhat disappointing because students do not perceive themselves as decision makers and they are influenced by social desirability.

Valiga, T. M. (1983). Cognitive development: A critical component of baccalaureate nursing education. *Image: The Journal of Nursing Scholarship, 15*, 115–119.

> A study to describe the cognitive development of freshman, sophomore, junior, and senior baccalaureate nursing students and to describe the change in cognitive development that occurred over the span of an academic year. Cognitive development was defined as the students' general structuring of knowledge and experience as measured by the Kre Wi instrument, a test employing a projective technique and essay questions to provide subjects with an opportunity to share their thinking about and processing of a subject.

25

Nursing Graduates

Arnold, J. M. (1985). *Diagnostic reasoning protocols for nursing clinical simulations*. Paper presented at the Measurement of Clinical and Nursing Outcomes Conference, New Orleans, Louisiana.

This report looked at both the process of diagnostic reasoning and the outcomes using a 126-item criterion reference questionnaire relative to a simulation. Indicators were observation, inference making, and decision making. The report concluded that nurses have difficulty deciding upon appropriate data for decisions.

Baumann, A., & Bourbonnais, F. (1982). Nursing decision making in critical areas. *Journal of Advanced Nursing, 7*, 435–446.

This is an exploratory study attempting to identify factors that critical care nurses consider relevant in making rapid patient care decisions. Using a semistructured interview, 50 critical care nurses were surveyed. The findings suggest that experience and knowledge are the most important factors influencing rapid decision making.

Carnevali, D. L., Mitchell, P. H., Woods, N. F., & Tauner, C. A. (1984). *Diagnostic reasoning in nursing*. Philadelphia: Lippencott.

This book discusses the general recognition of nursing's unique domain in health care and the clinician's rigorous, effective, and consistent use of the diagnostic reasoning process. This process is shown in application in a purely nursing perspective. Outcome evaluation is illustrated by use of computer simulation exercises and strategies for self-monitoring throughout professional growth.

Chastain, B. B. (1986). Zone of indifference: Effective decision making in critical care management. *Nursing Management, 17*(1), 34A–34E.

The author describes a zone of indifference toward position responsibilities and patients that can markedly interfere with decision making in the critical care area. It is suggested that through incentives and trust in the organization, the critical care nurse will be able to contribute to the organization in a productive and satisfying manner.

del Bueno, D. J. (1983). Doing the right thing: Nurses' ability to make clinical decisions. *Nurse Educator, 8*(3), 7–11.

Research article describes the evaluation of effectiveness of simulations developed to teach and assess nurses' clinical decision-making skills. The simulations, a series of videotaped patient situations, provides opportunity for participants to identify the nature of the patient problem and decide on a course of nursing action.

Ehrat, K. S. (1983). A model for politically astute planning and decision making. *The Journal of Nursing Administration, 13*(9), 29–35.

> The author discusses the administrative role in nursing service and edu cation. The role demands political interfaces in negotiations, conflicts, competition, and power struggles for scarce resources. It is suggested that the requisite skill to deal with such situations is a function of both organizational and career experiences. A model is presented to provide nurse administrators with a framework for appropriate planning and making the right decisions.

Grier, M. R. (1976). Decision making about patient care. *Nurse Research, 25*(2), 105–110.

> Four patient situations and a schedule of nursing actions and outcomes were presented to 47 registered nurses to investigate quantification of 185 nursing decisions about patient care. The expected value was calculated for all action outcomes. The findings suggested that decision theory is applicable to nursing and that nursing decisions can be adapted to analytical models.

Hansen, A. C., & Thomas, D. B. (1968). A conceptualization of decision making. *Nurse Research, 17*(5), 436–443.

> The purpose of the study was to report an analysis of the priority-for-home-visiting decision responses determined by public health nurses, using a framework developed for decision making. The schematic representation consisted of the situational, contextual, and decision maker variables which result in a decision response. Response varied by role group assignment.

Jenkins, H. M. (1985). Improved clinical decision-making in nursing. *Journal of Nursing Education, 24*(6), 242–243.

> The article suggested that teaching effective decision making is an attitude on the part of the teacher that allows the learner to fully experience the process of making decisions and being held accountable for them. It is emphasized that students must perceive themselves as capable of making clinical decisions in order to do so effectively.

Kelly, K. (1966). Clinical inference in nursing. I. A nurse's viewpoint. *Nursing Research, 15*(1), 23–26.

> The purpose of this research was to investigate the process of clinical inference with special reference to nursing. Phase I used a sign-symptoms/action data base to provide a representative situational basis for the study of cue-utilization by the nurse in the inference process. Phase II made an analysis of cue-utilization by the nurse. Phase III looked at the extent to which the nurse selects and reviews cues. Among results, it was suggested

that the complexity involved in the decision process makes it difficult to adhere to a predictable mathematical model.

Kostopoulos, M. R. (1985, June). *The reliability and validity of a registered nurse performance evaluation tool.* Paper presented at the Measurement of Clinical and Nursing Outcomes Conference, New Orleans, Louisiana.

> The paper reported on the establishment of reliability and validity for a criterion-referenced tool measuring nurse performance by observation using a Likert-like scale to be completed by the immediate supervisor. Specific expectations were stated in behavioral terms. It was concluded that further refinement is necessary to establish more acceptable reliability and validity.

McKay, P. S. (1983). Interdependent decision making: Redefining professional autonomy. *Nursing Administration Quarterly,* 7(4), 21–30.

> The author suggests that in light of the increasing amount of high technology used to provide patient care, professional health care practice is now a collective enterprise. Therefore, a redefinition of professional autonomy should include both independent and interdependent practice-related decision making as well as shared accountability.

Phillips, L. R., & Rempusheski, V. F. (1985). A decision-making model for diagnosing and intervening in elder abuse and neglect. *Nursing Research, 34*(3), 134–139.

> A grounded theory technique was used to develop a four-stage decision-making model for use in decisions involving neglectful and abusive relationships in the elderly. Complexity of decision processes is revealed through five alternative pathways through the model. It is concluded that the model would be useful in assisting health care providers to make better decisions about intervening in situations where elders are cared for by relatives in a home setting.

Sparks, R. K. (1982). Problem-solving ability of graduates from associate and baccalaureate degree nursing programs. *Journal of Nursing Education, 21*(8), 68–69.

> Problem-solving ability was measured using two self-report measures—Nursing Performance Simulation Instrument and Nursing Process Utilization Inventory—as well as demographic data. It was concluded that the use of the nursing process differs according to nursing preparation.

Taylor, A. G. (1978). Decision making in nursing: An analytical approach. *Journal of Nursing Administration, 8*(2), 22–30.

> Using the Vroom and Yelton decision model, four nursing situations are presented and analyzed by use of decision rules and diagnostic questions.

It is suggested that this model would be useful in assisting nurse-managers to improve their decision-making behavior.

Verhonick, P. J., Nichols, G. A., Glor, B. A. K., & McCarthy, R. T. (1968). I came, I saw, I responded: Nursing observation and action survey. *Nursing Research, 17,* 38–44.

> Five filmed patient simulations were viewed and survey responses on data cards were recorded by 1,965 individuals. The purpose of the survey was to gain insight into the type of observations made by nurses and the actions taken based on those observations. The authors suggested that results were inconclusive; however, it would appear that years of active nursing experience and highest degree held were important determinants of actions and observations.

Werly, H. H., & Grier, M. R. (1981). *Nursing information systems.* New York: Springer-Verlag.

> The authors emphasize the centrality of decision making to nursing practice and discuss the vital elements for making nursing decisions. They suggest that nurses have difficulty in acquiring and processing information for making decisions and definitively outline several organized, comprehensive approaches for establishing nursing diagnosis and for choosing appropriate interventions. It is emphasized that measurable patient/client outcomes should be an integral part of any process.

Non-nursing

Barrows, H. S., & Tamblyn, R. M. (1976). An evaluation of problem-based learning in small groups, utilizing a simulated patient. *Journal of Medical Education, 51,* 52–54.

> This study examined patient problem definition as an outcome of medical education using assessment skills, inquiry techniques, and peer consultation as various methods. Evaluation was conducted by self-report, essay examination of observations, and multiple-choice tests relevant to each simulation. Although no value was reported the study stated that interrater reliability was established for student formulations.

Einarson, T. R., McGhan, W. F., & Bootman, J. L. (1985). Decision analysis applied to pharmacy practice. *American Journal of Hospital Pharmacy, 42,* 364–371.

> The value of decision analysis in pharmacy practice is discussed because it encourages the practitioner to define views explicitly and to weigh the merits of each alternative. The potential outcome can be assessed by using a decision tree with the probability of occurrence of each choice indicated. A limitation is that probabilities are often estimated on the basis of the decision maker's biases.

Feinstein, E., Gustavson, L. P., & Levine, H. G. (1983). Measuring the instructional validity of clinical simulation problems. *Evaluation and the Health Professions, 6*(1), 61–76.

> Description of research in which written clinical simulation problems in forced-choice and essay formats were used to compare the performance of medical students with varying levels of clinical experience at the conclusion of their pediatric rotations. Clinical simulation problems failed to demonstrate responsiveness to development and maturation in the problem-solving approach to patient care.

Hill, P. H. (1979). *Making decisions: A multidisciplinary approach.* Reading, Massachusetts: Addison-Wesley.

> This volume provides the individual with several decision-making techniques, methods, and points of view. It uses a multidisciplinary approach that includes economics, engineering design, political science, and psychology. The book is intended to teach skill in decision making to an audience with no prior background in the discipline. The case study method is used to introduce concepts dealing with all aspects of the decision-making process. Self-evaluation is suggested.

Keely, S. M., Browne, M. N., & Kreutzer, J. S. (1982). A comparison of freshmen and seniors on general and specific essay tests of critical thinking. *Research in Higher Education, 17*(2), 139–154.

> This study used a series of specific open-ended questions and a single broad essay question to investigate the critical thinking abilities of freshmen and seniors. One hundred forty-five freshmen and 155 seniors participated in the study. The students were randomly assigned to take the General Questions Condition or the Specific Questions Condition. Each condition had two different essays, with a total of four essays to be evaluated. The rater was a graduate student trained in the scoring procedures by the authors. A second rater experienced in scoring critical thinking essays provided a check of interrater agreement. An overall correlation of .90 was established (there were variations among the different categories). ACT Composite scores were used as the covariates in two-way MANOVAs. The results showed that the seniors did surpass the freshmen but the absolute differences were not very large. The overall scores were low both for the freshmen and seniors, indicating a need for more direct training in critical thinking skills.

Montgomery, H., & Adelbratt, T. (1982). Gambling decisions and information about expected value. *Organizational Behavior and Human Performance, 29*, 39–57.

> This study looked at risk-taking behaviors in the form of gambling decisions with expected utility and expected value as indicators. The results of

the self-report questionnaire indicated that subjects preferred concrete information for decision making with a concrete pattern of features.

McGuire, C., & Babbett, D. (1967). Simulation technique in the measurement of problem-solving skills. *Journal of Educational Measurement, 4,* 1–10.

> Simulation technique is used in a series of branched problems in patient management requiring sequential analysis and decision. The problems are designed to measure aspects of behavior defined by a criterion group as essential components of clinical competence.

Mevarech, L. R., & Werner, S. (1985). Are mastery learning strategies beneficial for developing problem-solving skills? *Higher Education, 14,* 425–432.

> The purpose of this study was to compare three instructional methods for developing problem-solving skills in a paramedical course. The three instructional methods used were: Frontal Lecture Strategies (FLS), Mastery Learning Strategies (MLS, based on the belief that all students can attain high levels of achievement when instruction provides for individual differences in ability, rate, and other factors) and Experimental Mastery Learning Strategies (EMLS, modified MLS with specific experiential activities tailored to the problems encountered in the course). Problem-solving skills were assessed in three ways: (1) responses to a film and specific questions, (2) case study reports and (3) end-of-semester examinations with 25 lower mental processes and 25 higher mental processes questions. Scores were derived for all three measures, a MANOVA was performed, along with a series of ANOVAs with the three treatment groups. The findings indicated that the Experimental Mastery Learning Strategies group performed better on the measures of problem-solving skills, while the Frontal Lectures produced a stronger showing of the lower mental processes subscales.

Pennings, J. M. (1983). *Decision making: An organizational behavior approach.* New York: Markus Wiener Publishing, Inc.

> This is a collection of readings that looks at individual, organizational, and strategic areas of research in corporate decision making. Realizing that individuals make decisions about alternative plans and courses of action, suggestions are made for designing a work environment that is optimal for both the organization and the individual.

Rubin, T. I. (1985). *Overcoming indecisiveness.* New York: Harper and Row.

> The author outlines eight stages of effective decision making in this self-help book. Describing the difference between those willing to make an emotional investment and those who abdicate from such a process, he sug-

gests that knowledge of the process will facilitate utilization of it. Effectiveness is monitored by self-analysis.

Svenson, O. (1979). Process descriptions of decision making. *Organizational Behavior and Human Performance, 23*, 86–112.

> The paper introduces a representation system for the description of decision alternatives and decision rules, classified according to their metric requirements. It is suggested that most decision problems are solved without complete information and that many algebraic models of decision making are inadequate.

Taylor, R. N., & Dunnette, M. D. (1974). Relative contribution of decision-maker attributes to decision processes. *Organizational Behavior and Human Performance, 12*, 286–298.

> The article reports on a classic study looking at the outcomes of the decision-making process. Using a self-report questionnaire and two forms of the Personnel Decision Simulations, the study looked at executives' ability to make decisions and their outcomes based on sixteen demographic and psychological attributes including fourteen scales measuring the psychological attributes of intelligence. The authors concluded that outcomes of the process depend on such criteria as amount of information, processing rate, and decision confidence, accuracy, and flexibility.

Wright, G. (1984). *Behavioral decision theory: An introduction.* Beverly Hills, CA: Sage.

> This book deals primarily with individual decision making, focusing on four major issues: (1) how good are we at making decisions?; (2) can decision making be improved?; (3) how do we actually make decisions?; and (4) are some people better at making decisions than others? Based on a psychological perspective, the authors advocate constant self-monitoring and analysis techniques for measuring the effectiveness of decision making.

Nursing

Crisham, P. (1981). Measuring moral judgement in nursing dilemmas. *Nursing Research, 30*, 104–110.

> The purpose of the study was to (1) identify recurrent moral dilemmas experienced by staff nurses; (2) develop the Nursing Dilemma Test (NDT) to measure nurses' responses to nursing dilemmas and the importance given to moral issues and practical considerations; (3) relate staff nurses' responses to nursing dilemmas in the NDT and responses to hypothetical moral dilemmas in the Defining Issues Test to two variables of levels of nursing education and length of clinical experience; and (4) compare moral judgments of five subject groups (staff nurses with associate degrees, staff nurses with baccalaureate degrees, nurses with master's degrees in nursing, college junior pre-nurses and graduate level non-nurses).

Ketefian, S. (1981). Critical thinking, educational preparation and development of moral judgement among selected groups of practicing nurses. *Nursing Research, 30*(2), 98–103.

> A descriptive study of the relationship between critical thinking, educational preparation, and level of moral judgement in 79 practicing nurses of diploma, associate degree, baccalaureate, and higher educational backgrounds. The Watson–Glaser Critical Thinking Appraisal Test was used to measure critical thinking and Rest's Defining Issues Test was used to measure moral judgement.

Ketefian, S. (1981). Moral reasoning and moral behavior among selected group of practicing nurses. *Nursing Research, 30*(3), 171–176.

> Study examined the relationship between moral reasoning and moral behavior in 79 practicing nurses of diploma, associate degree, and baccalaureate educational backgrounds. Moral reasoning was measured by Rest's Defining Issues Test. Judgement about nursing decisions developed by the author was used to measure two components of moral behavior: knowledge and evaluation of ideal moral behavior and perception of realistic moral behavior.

Mayberry, M. A. (1986). Ethical decision-making: A response of hospital nurses. *Nursing Administration Quarterly, 10*(3), 75–81.

> This is a report of a study conducted to determine whether the levels of moral reasoning in ethical dilemmas of staff nurses and head nurses showed a relationship to level of preparation in nursing education, length of nursing experience, age, and size of employing agency. Results indicated that nurses more often use an intuitive approach to problem solving; staff nurses with baccalaureate preparation used the principled reasoning approach more than head nurses and other staff nurses with less academic training. The data also suggests that as nurses grow older and gain more experience, they become imbued with the organization's aim and develop loyalty to the institution and peers, factors which might serve as barriers to personal ethical decision making.

Non-nursing

Biggs, D. A., & Barnett, R. (1981). Moral judgement development of college students. *Research in Higher Education, 14*(2), 91–102.

> Four hundred seven freshman students agreed to participate in this study. They were all asked to complete the Defining Issues Test. The top 25 percent (N = 101) and the bottom 25 percent (N = 101) were selected to continue in the study and were asked to complete the Inventory of College Experiences, a measure of causal attribution, a measure of punitiveness, and a number of questions about their social and academic background. Three years later the students were asked to answer the same questionnaires. Forty-four students in the top group and 39 in the bottom group had usable data. Results of multiple regression analysis showed that different experiential, background, and attitude factors influence the level of moral judgement development of upper-division students.

Schlaefli, A., Rest, J. R., & Thoma, S. J. (1985). Does moral education improve moral judgement? A meta-analysis of intervention studies using the defining issues test. *Review of Educational Research, 55*(3), 319–352.

> This is a meta-analysis of 55 studies of educational interventions designed to stimulate development of moral judgement. Subject groups included junior and senior high school students and college and graduate students 24 years of age or older.

Sheehan, T. J., Candee, D., Willms, J., Donnelly, J. C., & Husted, S. D. (1985). Structural equation models of moral reasoning and physician performance. *Evaluation and the Health Professions, 8*(4), 379–400.

> To identify and explain aspects of clinical performance related to moral reasoning 39 family medicine residents were (1) observed via videotape as

they interacted with each of two simulated patients and (2) interviewed to assess the performance with each patient, elicit their general philosophy of being a doctor, and measure their moral reasoning. Structural models were developed to explicate the relationship between moral reasoning performance on simulated cases, performance as a resident, attitude and intention.

6 PROFESSIONAL ATTITUDES AND SOCIALIZATION

Nursing

Cassells, J. M., Redman, B. K., & Jackson, S. S. (1986). Student choice of baccalaureate nursing programs, their perceived level of growth and development, career plans, and transition into practice. *Journal of Professional Nursing, 2*(3), 186–196.

> A descriptive survey of 1985 senior nursing students just prior to graduation was conducted to ascertain perceptions about baccalaureate nursing education as preparation for a professional nursing career. A follow-up survey was conducted six months following graduation. Most 1985 graduate participants felt prepared for their first clinical position, reporting that they frequently applied therapeutic communication principles, nursing diagnosis, and nursing process in their practice. Appropriate comparisons are made to respondents of the 1984 project.

Cotanch, P. H. (1981). Self-actualization and professional socialization of nursing students in the clinical laboratory experience. *Journal of Nursing Education, 20*(8), 4–14.

> This study compared junior and senior nursing students on their scores on the Shostroms Personal Orientation Inventory and the investigator designed Clinical Student Perception Questionnaire.

Dagenais, F., & Meleis, A. I. (1982). Professionalism, work ethics, and empathy in nursing: The nurse self-description form. *Western Journal of Nursing Research, 4*(4), 407–422.

> This scale was originally developed for use in studying creative performance among National Aeronautic and Space Administration scientists and engineers. The instrument was adapted and validated for nurses by a group of WCHEN researchers and used to measure the effectiveness of a leadership course. The authors explored the possibility of using this form to identify several subscales. The form has 19 items and the authors identified 3 subscales (professionalism, work ethic, and empathy).

Dear, M. R., & Kien, M. F. (1982). Role transition: A practicum for baccalaureate nursing students. *Journal of Nursing Education, 21*(2), 32–37.

> This article discusses a role transition course for senior nursing students. Evaluation methods were a philosophy of nursing paper, journal entries, care plans, the Slater Nursing Competencies Rating Scale, and self-evaluation.

Kramer, M., Polifroni, E. C., & Organek, N. (1986). Effects of faculty practice on student learning outcomes. *Journal of Professional Nursing, 2,* 289–301.

> A study of the relationship between faculty practice and student acquisition of beliefs, values, and attributes associated with professional craftsmanship. For a sample of 134 baccalaureate senior nursing students the variables of autonomy, locus of control, self-concept, and self-esteem, professional and bicultural role behavior, and characteristics associated with the professional role were measured using Levinson's Perception of Events, the nurse self-concept instrument, the role behavior instrument, the Pankratz tool to measure autonomy, and a tool devised to measure the construct of professional craftsmanship.

Lawler, T. G. (1985). *Measuring socialization to the professional role.* Paper presented at the Measurement of Clinical and Nursing Outcomes Conference, New Orleans, Louisiana.

> The study looked at the outcome of nursing education at both the associate level and the baccalaureate level generic program. The author favored Stone's Health Care Professional Attitude Inventory, as revised by Lawler, as a measurement of professional orientation to nursing. It was stated that the comparative tool, Corwin's Nursing Role Conception Scale had questionable value because of the emphasis on professional role deprivation or dissonance.

Little, M., & Brian, S. (1982). The challengers, interactors, and mainstreamers: Second-step education and nursing roles. *Nursing Research, 31,* 239–245.

> A factor analysis of longitudinal data obtained using the Omnibus Personality Inventory (OPI) and two questionnaires developed by the National Second-Step Project for 236 nursing students in six second-step programs. Funding indicated students entering these programs varied greatly in professional attitudes. At graduation students perceived themselves as more professionally involved, committed and competent, but they did not change similarly in other areas of life.

Lynn, M. R. (1981). *The professional socialization of nursing students: A comparison based on types of educational programs.* Paper presented at the annual meeting of the American Educational Research Associations, Los Angeles, CA. (ERIC Document Reproduction Service No. ED 201 268).

Two new scoring methods for the Nurses Professional Orientation Scale (NPOS) were developed and tested on associate (N = 120) and baccalaureate (N = 156) senior nursing students in order to advance the assessment of professional socialization. Scoring methods were based on (1) traditional versus nontraditional views of nursing and (2) practicing nurses' views on nursing.

McCain, N. L. (1985). A test of Cohen's developmental model for professional socialization with baccalaureate nursing students. *Journal of Nursing Education, 24*(5), 180–185.

This study was designed to test the Cohen model of professional socialization. This model proposes that nursing students progress through four developmental stages of unilateral dependence, negative/independence, dependence/mutuality, and interdependence as they advance through an educational program.

Meleis, A., & Farrell, K. D. (1974). A study of senior students in three nursing programs. *Nursing Research, 23*(6), 461–468.

One hundred eighty-eight students in three programs (diploma, associate, and baccalaureate) were tested to determine whether graduates of different programs present a different quality of nursing care.

Murray, L. A., & Morris, D. R. (1982). Professional autonomy among senior nursing students in diploma, associate degree, and baccalaureate nursing programs. *Nursing Research, 31*, 311–313.

This study attempts to compare the degree of professional autonomy among senior nursing students (N = 224) from a diploma, an associate degree, and a baccalaureate program using the Pankratz Nursing Questionnaire. Significant differences among the means for three programs were found for the autonomy, patients rights, and rejection of the traditional nursing role limitations subscales.

Overfield, T., & Duffy, M. E. (1984). Research on teaching research in the baccalaureate nursing curriculum. *Journal of Advanced Nursing, 9*, 189–196.

This paper reviewed the research literature on teaching research to undergraduate nursing students. There are only five formal research studies that address specific questions regarding the teaching of research. Three of these studies were surveys of schools of nursing; two were evaluations and descriptions of more specific courses. The authors recommend more research in the area of determining which method or combination of methods educates nurses to read and use research findings in their practice. The authors suggest the use of the Thomas Price inventory to measure the attitudes of students and their knowledge of research.

Sakalys, J. A. (1984). Effects of an undergraduate research course on cognitive development. *Nursing Research, 33*(5), 290–295.

> The purpose of this study was to examine the effects of a research methods course on undergraduate nursing students' cognitive development or reflective judgement level. The sample was composed of 50 senior female nursing students who volunteered to participate in this study. One-half (the experimental group) were enrolled in the required research course, while the other half (the control group) were planning to enroll in the research course the subsequent semester. All subjects were asked to complete the Reflective Judgement Interview which was designed to ascertain the students' stage of cognitive development. This measure differentiates seven levels of cognitive development, with levels six and seven judged to be the level at which a person is ready to propose and conduct research.

Swenson, I., & Kleinbaum, A. (1984). Attitudes toward research among undergraduate nursing students. *Journal of Nursing Education, 23*(9), 380–386.

> The purpose of this study was to determine if there was an attitudinal change about research among undergraduate nursing students during their two years in a baccalaureate nursing program. An attitude questionnaire designed by the investigators and a future career plans questionnaire also designed by the investigators were administered to the students as a pretest in the first junior class, as a posttest at the end of the first junior semester, and as a posttest at the end of the first senior semester.

Tetreault, A. I. (1976). Selected factors associated with professional attitude of baccalaureate nursing students. *Nursing Research, 25*(1), 49–53.

> Eight hypotheses were tested to examine the association between professional attitude and selected situational and demographic factors of baccalaureate nursing students.

Weiss, S. J. (1984). The effect of transition modules on new graduate adaptation. *Research in Nursing and Health, 7*, 51–59.

> The purpose of this study was to determine the effectiveness of educational modules for new graduate nurses adapting to the work setting. Each new graduate was given Corwin's Role Conception Scale, Suman's Powerlessness Scale, Benner's Clinical Skills Inventory, and Munson's Job Satisfaction Index.

Non-nursing Students

Dietrich, M. C., & Doran, R. L. (1978). Work values contrasts at the associate and baccalaureate student levels in the medical laboratory services. *Evaluation and the Health Professions, 1*(4), 217–227.

> Research study to examine the work values pattern in male and female students at the associate and baccalaureate levels of medical laboratory sciences profession. Responses from 320 students on Super's Work Value Inventory led to the conclusion that the two-year students placed greater emphasis on extrinsic values related to work outcomes and that a student's educational level or sex has an impact on his or her work orientation.

Pace, R. (1984). *Measuring the quality of college student experiences.* Los Angeles: University of California.

> The book provides details about the College Student Experience Questionnaire including format, content, and address for ordering. The instrument includes valid and reliable scales for measuring quality of effort. Use of these measures has increased understanding of and provided explanations for college student learning and development.

7 SATISFACTION

Nursing

Cassells, J. M., Redman, B., & Jackson, S. S. (1986). Generic baccalaureate nursing student satisfaction regarding professional and personal development prior to graduation and one year post graduation. *Journal of Professional Nursing, 2*, 114–127.

> A report from the Generic Baccalaureate Nursing Data project in which full-time baccalaureate senior students not holding RN licenses were surveyed regarding their satisfaction with their development during their nursing program and then surveyed again one year after graduation to ascertain their choice of jobs, satisfaction with job-related factors, and involvement in patient care decisions.

Cornell, G. R. (1985). *Measures of nursing students' satisfaction as related to selected proxy measures of quality education at the North East Missouri State University—the added value approach.* Paper presented at the Measurement of Clinical and Nursing Outcomes Conference, New Orleans, Louisiana.

> The author developed a norm-referenced measure for nursing student satisfaction with the university program using class, sex, and professional socialization as predictors. It was concluded that these criteria explained only 26 percent of the variance.

Non-nursing

Hearn, J. C. (1985). Determinants of college students' overall evaluation of their academic programs. *Research in Higher Education, 23*(4), 413–437.

> Research study explored the determinants of college seniors' overall evaluations of their academic programs. The sample consisted of 775 students at two universities in the early 1970s. Findings suggest stimulating coursework and good teaching were somewhat more important than opportunities for faculty/student interaction or perceived faculty knowledgeability. However, faculty availability and course stimulations were

more critical among women than men. Theoretical and applied implications are discussed. The study includes numerous tables of statistical findings.

Hendel, D. (1985). Effects of individualized and structured college curricula on students' performance and satisfaction. *American Educational Research Journal, 22,* 117–122.

> Study to compare the effects of individualized and structured curricula on the academic performance and follow-up satisfaction of 428 students who applied for admission to an individualized degree university program. Results of the randomized experiment indicated the two groups did not differ significantly in persistence, graduation rate, academic success, and overall course selection patterns but did differ significantly in their evaluation of their graduate education at follow-up.

Smart, J. C., & Ethington, C. A. (1985). Early career outcomes of baccalaureate recipients: A study of native four-year and transfer two-year college students. *Research in Higher Education, 22,* 185–193.

> Study explores differences in the job status, job stability, and job satisfaction of 1,609 baccalaureate recipients in 1976 (who were participants in the National Longitudinal Study of the high school class of 1972) with varying lengths of attendance at two-year institutions. Results of the multivariate analysis of covariance of the data indicated no significant difference in job stability, status, or satisfaction of (male and female) transfer two-year college and native four-year college baccalaureate recipients during the early years of their careers when variations associated with their initial levels of academic ability, family, socioeconomic status, and intended occupational status are statistically controlled.

Nursing Students

Ellis, L. (1980). An investigation of nursing student self-concept levels: A pilot study. *Nursing Research, 29*(6), 389–390.

> The Tennessee Self-Concept Scale was administered to all four classes of a baccalaureate program to determine if any differences in self-concept existed between the four levels.

George, T. B. (1982). Development of the self-concept of nurse in nursing students. *Research in Nursing and Health, 5*, 191–197.

> A descriptive cross-sectional study to determine if components of nursing students' self-concepts change as they progress through their educational program. For a sample of 132 generic nursing students of one baccalaureate program chi-square analysis of responses to the Twenty Statements Test indicated no significant difference in self-concept by grade level (sophomore, junior, and senior) in the number of primary nursing references.

Goldstein, J. O. (1980). Comparison of graduating AD and baccalaureate nursing students' characteristics. *Nursing Research, 29*, 46–49.

> A study to investigate differences in self-actualization between AD graduating nursing students (N = 159) and baccalaureate graduating nursing students (N = 204) as measured by scores on the Personal Orientation Inventory in time competence/incompetence, outer/inner ratio, valuing (self-actualizing value and existentiality), feeling (reactivity and spontaneity), self-perception (self-regard and self-acceptance), synergistic awareness (perception of the nature of man and synergy), and interpersonal sensitivity (acceptance of aggression and capacity for intimate contact).

Olson, R. K., Gesley, R. S., & Heater, B. S. (1984). The effects of undergraduate clinical internship on the self-concept and professional role mastery of baccalaureate nursing students. *Journal of Nursing Education, 23*, 105–108.

> Study to determine whether an eight-week undergraduate clinical course would enhance students' self-concepts and increase their percep-

45

tion of competence in critical care teaching/collaboration, planning/ evaluation, professional development, leadership, and interpersonal skills and communication. A pretest—posttest design using the Tennessee Self-Concept Scale and the Six Dimensional Scale of Nursing Performance was utilized for the study.

Stevens, K. R. (1983). The relation of locus of control, sex-role identity, and assertiveness in baccalaureate students. *Dissertation Abstracts International, 43,* 3539B.

The aim of this study was to increase the understanding of the interrelationships among the aspects of personal control, sex role identity, and assertiveness in nursing students. The objectives were to (1) describe the profiles of locus of control, sex role identity, and assertiveness of beginning and graduating nursing students and (2) describe how these attributes are related to the nursing student population. The measures used were (1) the Levenson locus of control scale to measure internal control, powerful others, and chance, (2) the Personal Attributes Questionnaire to measure sex role identity, and (3) the Rathus Assertiveness Schedule. "Reliability of the instruments was moderate to high." Graduating students scored significantly higher on assertiveness than the beginning students. Locus of control and sex role identity were minimally related; both are necessary for a comprehensive explanation of assertiveness.

Non-nursing

Colditz, G. A., & Sheenan, M. (1982). The impact of instructional style on the development of professional characteristics. *Medical Education, 16,* 127–132.

This study examined the extent to which the educational environment of individual subjects, distinct from their educational content, affected the acquisition of attitudes, behaviors, and cognitive skills. Faculty identified 15 attitudinal and behavioral characteristics which they considered important in a competent medical practitioner. Characteristics were classified according to cognitive and learning styles, empathic and interpersonal skills, and professional and ethical qualities. First year students completed the questionnaire, identifying whether specific courses/subjects encouraged, discouraged, or did neither for the 15 attitudinal and behavioral characteristics. The study supported greater emphasis on structure rather than content in curriculum. An increase in independent learning and self-education was recommended. Also recommended were integration of learning rather than specialist isolation and greater delegation of responsibility to the student for the selection, organization, and pacing of the knowledge to be learned.

Erskine, C. G., Westerman, G. H., & Grandy, T. G. (1986). Personality styles of first-year dental students. *Journal of Dental Education, 50*, 221–224.

> The Meyers Briggs Type Indicator (MBTI) was used to measure the personality styles of dental students in two first-year classes. The implications for the organization and curriculum of dental schools considering the personality traits of these dental students are described.

Reeve, P. E., & Watson, C. J. (1985). An exploration of the attitudes, personality, and performance of dental students. *Medical Education, 19*, 226–237.

> This study investigates the behavioral patterns, performance, and attitudes to dentistry and the personality traits in male and female dental students studying at the Cardiff Dental School in Wales. Certain characteristics in dental students which were predictors of success were identified and could be useful for initial selection or entry into the field. Instruments used included a questionnaire about curriculum and Catell's personality inventory. The 16 PFQ Form C results were correlated with students' "A" level grades, interview grades, clinical examination results, and response to some items of the general questionnaire. The study found no consistent relationship between intelligence and performance nor between "A" level results and the bachelor of dental surgery exam.

Robbins, L., Robbins, E. S., Katz, S. E., Geliebter, B., & Stern, M. (1983). Achievement motivation in medical students. *Journal of Medical Education, 58*, 850–858.

> The study was designed to assess similarities and differences between male and female, third- and fourth-year medical students in three major areas: fear of success; interests and attitudes toward medical school; and expectations concerning combining future career with family life responsibilities. Instruments used were projective techniques developed by Horner, the Strong Interest Inventory, and an attitude questionnaire.

9 GENERAL INFORMATION ON EDUCATIONAL OUTCOMES

Specific to Nursing

American Association of Colleges of Nursing. (1986). *Essentials of college and university education for nursing, a working document. Washington, DC: Author.*

> This project was developed to define the essentials of college and university education for nursing. The idea for the project came from several recommendations in the Institute of Medicine Study on Nursing and Nursing Education (1983) and Report of the National Commission on Nursing (1983). Three work groups focused on the following areas: (1) essential knowledge, (2) essential skilled practice, and (3) essential attitudes and personal qualities.

Clark, N., & Smith, D. (1984). *North Dakota statewide nursing study, phase II, delineation of nursing practice.* Bismark, ND: North Dakota State Board of Nursing. (ERIC Document Reproduction Service No. 260 664)

> Two hundred fifty-three-page research report which is part of a larger study concerning (1) scope of nursing practice; (2) specific competencies currently targeted by nursing education; (3) differences in specific competencies endorsed by nurses with various education preparations as observed by nurses within the state; and (4) employers' observations of minimum education preparation required for performance of the competencies. The report includes numerous appendices (including the Nursing Delineation Surveys).

Clark, N., & Smith, D. (1984). *North Dakota statewide nursing study, phase III, final report and recommendations.* Bismark, ND: North Dakota State Board of Nursing. (ERIC Document Reproduction Service No. 260 665)

> The process, outcomes, and recommendations resulting from a project to develop a statewide nursing resource planning system. One of the five outcomes of the project was a delineation of nursing practice that provided a base for curriculum development/revision for the different levels of nursing education.

49

Coleman, E. (1986). On redefining the baccalaureate degree. *Nursing and Health Care, 7,* 193–196.

> In this paper the author describes a project sponsored by the Association of American Colleges (AAC) that explored the question of coherence and integrity in undergraduate education and proposed a minimum required curriculum. Criteria were identified for the required curriculum: (1) inquiry, abstract logical thinking, critical analysis; (2) literacy, writing, reading, speaking, listening; (3) understanding numerical data; (4) historical consciousness; (5) science; (6) values; (7) art; (8) international and multicultural experiences; and (9) study-in-depth.

Holzemer, W. L. (Ed.). (1986). *Review of research in nursing education, volume I.* New York: National League for Nursing.

> One hundred eighty-eight-page book provides an analytical review and synthesis of research conducted in nursing education. Topics were selected on the basis of availability of research to allow a review to be conducted. Topical areas include clinical judgement, professional socialization, clinical teaching, predictors of academic success, stress and the RN student, stress and critical care nursing, hospital staff development, and the clinical nurse specialist.

Johnson, J. J. (1985). *Assessment of students in relation to curriculum objectives and correlated with other data.* Paper presented at the Measurement of Clinical and Nursing Outcomes Conference, New Orleans, Louisiana.

> This paper dealt with the measurement of outcomes of nursing education, correlating self-report assessment and teacher observation, which were based on curriculum objectives, and various indicators of performance.

King, E. C. (1983). *Affective Education in Nursing: A Guide to Teaching and Assessment.* Queenstown, MD: Aspen Institute.

> The purpose of this book is to provide nursing instructors with strategies for preparing for classroom instruction and for evaluating it for the affective domain. The rationale for affective learning is discussed; the importance of developing individual skill in moral analysis and value clarification is emphasized; and a systematic approach in instructional design is suggested. Several teaching strategies are outlined. Four orientations to affective assessment are presented: (1) the psychometric, (2) the behavioral, (3) the counseling, and (4) the traditional approaches. Role-playing and simulation exercises are discussed in depth.

Lang, N. M., & Clinton, J. F. (1983). Assessment and assurance of the quality of nursing care. *Evaluation and the Health Professions, 6,* 211–231.

> This article reports empirical studies addressing structure, process, or outcome dimensions of nursing quality assurance. This is an overview for nursing care, but can also be used by educators. Six general outcome categories are presented: (1) physical health status outcome used by researchers, (2) mental health status, (3) social and physical functioning measures, (4) utilization of professional health resources, (5) health attitudes, knowledge, and behavior measures, and (6) patient perception of quality of nursing care.

Lenburg, C. B. (1984). An update on the regents external degree program. *Nursing Outlook, 32,* 250–254.

> Brief discussion of the program's history and current directions emphasizing collaborative efforts with other institutions to provide focused yet flexible learning for the nontraditional nursing student. Emphasizes specifically prescribed measurement of cognitive and performance outcomes at national networks of assessment centers as an essential component of the program.

MacLean, T. B., Knoll, G. H., & Kinney, C. K. (1985). The evaluation of a baccalaureate program for registered nurses. *Journal of Nursing Education, 24,* 53–57.

> The authors discuss ten years of experience with one RN-BSN program and describe procedures for advanced placement credit and special RN courses. Descriptive data and success measures of the 198 graduates of the original curriculum are presented as well as support systems and program changes that proved helpful.

Wise, P., & Cox, H. (1984). Evaluating a continuing nursing education program. *The Journal of Continuing Education in Nursing, 15*(4), 117–121.

> Report of an approach to programmatic evaluation using the Stakes model which includes information about the learners themselves, the antecedents (those things that existed prior to the learning event), the transactions (the learning process), the outcomes (behaviors the learners were expected to demonstrate), the procedure used, lines of communication, recommendations, and the evaluation process flow.

Not Limited to Nursing

Adelman, C. (1983). The major seventh: Standards as a leading tone in higher education. In J. R. Warren (Ed.), *Meeting the new demand for standards* (pp. 39–54). San Francisco, CA: Jossey-Bass.

> Cites recommendations by large employers for outcomes of education. These are the development of specific capacities, traits, and attitudes by colleges and universities for the sake of maintaining their own public standards for student learning and growth.

American Association of State Colleges and Universities. (1984). *In pursuit of degrees with integrity: A value-added approach to undergraduate assessment* (Report No. ISBN-0-88044-106-2). Washington, DC: Author. (ERIC Document Reproduction Service No. ED 251 036).

> One hundred two-page descriptive report of the Value-Added Program at Northeast Missouri State University. The report also includes five case studies. Appendices include information on assessment instruments and a questionnaire for students who are graduating.

Astin, A. (1979). Student-oriented management: A proposal for change. *Evaluating Education Quality: A Conference Summary of Washington Council on Postsecondary Accreditation, 3–18.*

> The author advocates the use of three "core" measures in evaluating educational objectives and outcomes: (1) successful completion of program of study, (2) cognitive development, and (3) student satisfaction.

Baird, L. (1985). Do grades and tests predict adult accomplishment? *Research in Higher Education, 23*(1), 3–85.

> A lengthy review of approximately 20 years (1966–1984) of studies relating accomplishment, achievement, or creativity with grades, academic ability, or test scores. Report includes extensive references.

Banta, T. W., & Fisher, H. S. (1984). *Performance funding: Tennessee's noble experiment in promoting program quality through assessment of outcomes.* Paper presented at the meeting of the American Educational Research Association, New Orleans, LA (ERIC Document Reproduction Service No. ED 247 842).

> Fifteen-page conference paper discusses the use of student outcome information at the University of Tennessee at Knoxville. Student outcomes studied included (1) achievement in general education, (2) achievement in the major field, and (3) opinion measurement concerning the quality of academic programs and services.

Billings, A. G., & Moos, R. H. (1982). Social support and functioning among community and clinical groups: A panel model. *Journal of Behavioral Medicine, 5*(3), 295–310.

> A longitudinal assessment of a representative sample of community men and women was conducted to examine the relationship between social support and personal functioning.

Bjorksten, O., Sutherland, S., Miller, C., & Stewart, T. (1983). Identification of medical students' problems and comparison with those of other students. *Journal of Medical Education, 58,* 759–767.

> In the study the perceived problems of medical students were compared with those of students in other health science colleges at the same institution.

Bowen, H. (1979, December). Outcomes assessment—A new era in accreditation. *The Proceedings of the Annual Convention of the Middle States Association of Colleges and Schools,* 27–38.

> The author recommends gathering of information to determine in what way students change. He identifies principles to be followed in the identification and evaluation of outcomes.

Bowen, H. (1977). *Investment in learning: The individual and social value of American higher education.* San Francisco, CA: Jossey-Bass.

> The author indicates the basic task is to modify the system of higher education so that it can continue to accommodate traditional students and to cultivate exceptional talent; and at the same time, to reach out to the new student of all ages whose educational needs, at least during a transitional phase, may be different from those of traditional students.

Boyle, A., & Santelli, J. (1986). Assessing the psychomotor skills: The role of the Crawford small parts dexterity test as a screening instrument. *Journal of Dental Education, 50,* 176–179.

> Longitudinal study designed to assess the validity of the CSPDT as a predictor of success in the psychomotor aspects of dental education, specifically the preclinical technique course.

Cornell, G. R. (1985). The value-added approach to the measurement of educational quality. *Journal of Professional Nursing, 1,* 356–363.

> This article describes the value-added approach to evaluating quality of education through objective and subjective measurement of student out-

comes. Undergraduates are tested at regularly scheduled intervals with nationally-normed examinations to gather objective data. Subjective data regarding student satisfaction with the nursing program, university, and support services are measured. A model of the application of the value-added approach within the nursing program is provided.

Dumont, R. G., & Troelstrup, R. L. (1980). Exploring relationships between objective and subjective measures of instructional outcomes. *Research in Higher Education, 12*(1), 37–51.

> This pilot study was conducted on a stratified random sample of 112 seniors at Tennessee Technological University and investigated the issue of construct validity of student testimony data as indicators of selected general educational outcomes. All students took four subtests of the ACT battery; 104 took the "Communicating" and "Problem Solving" portions of the ACT COMP (College Outcomes Measures Project). One month later 93 of the students completed a questionnaire in which they were asked to self-report their progress in the pursuit of 14 general educational goals.

Elfner, E. S., McLaughlin, R. K., Williamson, J. A., & Hardy, R. R. (1985, April/May). *Assessing goal-related student outcomes for academic decision making.* Paper presented at the Annual Forum of the Association for Institutional Research, Portland, OR. (ERIC Document Reproduction Service No. ED 259 669).

> Thirty-page research paper in which an input–output model for studying student outcomes is examined along with the results of a longitudinal study using this approach. Two survey tools were designed. Factor analysis resulted in 17 outcome variables concerning student satisfaction, perceptions of the college's contributions to intellectual development, personal goal development, self-image, and self-confidence.

Ewell, P. T. (1985). Assessment: What's it all about. *Change, 17*(6), 32–36.

> Institutional accountability in higher education and accountability based on measuring objective outcomes are described. Assessment, whether it can be performed objectively, and what effects external accountability pressures will have on the practices of higher education are discussed.

Ewell, P. T. (Ed.). (1985) *Assessing educational outcomes.* San Francisco, CA: Jossey-Bass.

> Provides numerous case studies—University of Tennessee, Knoxville (UTK), Northwest Missouri State University (NMSU), and Alverno College. Emphasizes that effective institutional assessment programs are team efforts.

Ewell, P. T. (1985). *The cost of assessment.* Paper presented at the National Conference on Assessment in Higher Education, Columbia, SC. (ERIC Document Reproduction Service No. ED 260 681).

> Forty-three-page conference paper addresses the unit of analysis and what to count as costs for assessment. Constructed cost estimates are provided for four typical institutions. Appendix includes brief descriptions and costs of commonly used commercial instruments for assessing student cognitive growth, reactions to college, and experiences after graduation.

Gluch-Scranton, J., & Gurenlian, J. (1985). A model for two-year and baccalaureate clinical dental hygiene education. *Journal of Dental Education, 49*, 95–99.

> This article examines the clinical role differentiation for dental hygienists and attempts to defend the position that differences should exist in clinical education within associate and baccalaureate degree programs. A model outlining distinguishing characteristics in clinical education for the associate and baccalaureate level is presented.

Guenike-Holl, L., Mentkowski, M., Much, N., Mertens, S., & Rogers, G. (1985, March). *Evaluating college outcomes through alumni studies: Measuring post college learning abilities.* Paper presented at annual meeting of the American Education Research Association, Chicago. (ERIC Document Reproduction Service No. ED 261 626).

> Thirty-four-page paper describing ongoing research of educational outcomes of graduates of Alverno College. Investigations included (1) expectations of college seniors and their goal achievements after graduation, (2) alumni evaluations of the relationship of their college preparation to goal achievement, (3) a comparison of career goals and decision making at the time of the senior year and after graduation, (4) whether alumni use abilities learned in college on the job, and (5) whether alumni continue learning and if self-sustained learning is evident at work.

Harcleroad, F. F., & Dickey, F. G. (1975). *Educational auditing and voluntary institutional accreditation.* Washington, DC: American Association of Higher Education.

> Recent court cases emphasize the nature of public accountability. Pressures may be building to the point where the inhouse function—improving individual institutions—though important, will become a secondary function. While accrediting agencies may continue to emphasize the improvement of member institutions as the primary purpose of their existence, the general public perceives the primary purpose of accreditation as certification of the level of quality of an institution or program. If this is the case, the accrediting agency takes on more of the characteristics of a

public regulatory commission with a responsibility for protecting the public. The agency becomes less oriented toward the membership and more
toward the public as a whole.

Harris, J. (1978). A new day in assessment in higher education. *Educational Record*, 268–282.

> The author explores the role that assessment of student performance could play as higher education tries to cope with trends of declining enroll-ments, competency-based curricula, accountability, and budgeting.

Harris, J. (1985). *Assessing outcomes in higher education: Practical suggestions for getting started*. Paper presented at the National Conference on Assessment in Higher Education, Columbia, SC. (ERIC Document Reproduction Service No. ED 260 677)

> Fifty-nine-page paper discussing the use of national and campus tests/measures to assess student academic achievement, attitudes, and be-havior. Externally-validated instruments are identified for the assessment of student performance in associate and baccalaureate programs in some fields. Publications, testing programs, and sources of information are also identified.

Huffman, J. (1982). The role of accreditation in preserving edu-cational integrity. *Educational Record*, 41–44.

> The author recommends that accrediting agencies motivate colleges and universities to pay more attention to the learning outcomes of their stu-dents.

Kirkwood, R. (1981). Process or outcomes—A false dichotomy. In T. M. Stauffer (Ed.), *Higher education's principal challenge* (pp. 63–68). Washington, DC: American Council on Education.

> Kirkwood provides a plan for measuring outcomes: (1) an evaluation of undergraduate scholastic achievement made by comparing scores on stan-dardized tests with the results on entrance placement exams; (2) a study of performance of graduates in senior colleges or in graduate and profes-sional schools; and (3) a long-term study of achievements (both vocational and avocational) of the alumni, based on data gathered periodically and systematically.

Kuh, G. (1981). *Indices of quality in the undergraduate experience*. Washington, DC: AAHE-ERIC/Higher Education Research Report, 4.

> Kuh cites outcome indices as measures of quality. These are persistence (rate of retention), achievement, intellectual and social emotional develop-ment, and alumni.

Kulik, J. A., Kulik, C. L. C., & Cohen, P. A. (1980). Effectiveness of computer-based college teaching: A meta-analysis of findings. *Review of Educational Research, 50*, 525–544.

> Presents a meta-analysis of findings from 59 evaluations of computer-based college teaching. Results indicated computer-based instruction made small but significant contributions to the course achievement and to attitudes toward instruction and subject matter. There were five major outcome types: student achievement, correlation between aptitude and achievement, course completion, student attitudes, and instructional time. Fifty-nine evaluation studies were completed from 1967 through 1978.

Lenning, O. T. (Ed.). (1976). *Improving educational outcomes.* San Francisco, CA: Jossey-Bass.

> One hundred-page volume explores the potential of various educational activities for improving student outcomes. The first three chapters are concerned with structuring the environment, structuring instructional process, and increasing learning in developmental education programs. Program effectiveness and related cost evaluation strategy at Empire State College are described. A comprehensive reference list is provided.

Lenning, O. T. (1977). *Previous attempts to structure educational outcomes and outcome-related concepts: A compilation and review of the literature.* Boulder, Colorado: National Center for Higher Education Management Systems.

> A 231-page literature review of (1) literature in the field of taxonomy for principles or criteria to be considered in developing an outcomes classification structure; (2) literature describing previous attempts at classifying educational outcomes and outcome-related concepts; and (3) literature on specific postsecondary-education outcomes that could be used to generate a broad list of outcomes for use in testing the National Center for Higher Education Management Systems (NCHEMS) Outcomes Structure. Many models are included throughout the book.

Lewis, J., & Nelson, K. (1983). The relationship between college grades and three factors of adult achievement. *Educational and Psychological Measurement, 43*, 577–580.

> Study of 575 graduates of one state university to determine the relationship of grades earned as undergraduates to three adult behaviors seen as relevant to the generalized goals of a liberal education: (1) quality of vocational achievement; (2) acceptance of responsibility in social groups; (3) further intellectual development. The only significant finding was an inverse relationship with involvement in community activities among males.

58   Chapter 9

Mentkowski, M., & Doherty, A. (1984). *Careering after college: Establishing the validity of ability learned in college for later careering and professional performance. Final report to the National Institute of Education. Overview and summary.* Milwaukee, WI: Alverno College. (ERIC Document Reproduction Service No. ED 252 144)

> The validity of skills developed in college to subsequent career performance was studied at Alverno College. Emphasis of the study was on whether competencies and assessment techniques of the learning process are valid; how students change on college outcomes; whether outcomes are mirrored in students' perceptions of their learning and abilities; how outcomes in college relate to lifelong learning; abilities, careering, and professional development after college; and the competencies that describe the performance and perceptions of outstanding professionals. Descriptions and validation studies of instruments are included.

Merwin, J. (1973). Educational measurement of what characteristics of whom (or what) by whom and why. *Journal of Educational Measurement, 10,* 1–6.

> Report indicates there is the need to work toward improvement in the quality of measures and measurement techniques available to meet information needs. The author offers several suggestions.

Millard, R. (1984). Assessing the quality of innovative graduate programs. In M. J. Pelczar, Jr., & L. C. Solomon (Eds.), *Keeping graduate programs responsive to national needs* (pp. 41–48). San Francisco, CA: Jossey-Bass.

> A specific, clear set of objectives of the program is necessary before effective quality assessment of the program can take place. There are a variety of conditions for the achievement of such objectives. Factors which have a direct bearing on the achievement of objectives include adequate resources, the relevance of faculty qualifications, and a commitment by the institution.

Olscamp, P. J. (1978). Can program quality be quantified? *Journal of Higher Education, 49,* 504–511.

> Three tasks in higher education: (1) quantitative accountability, (2) quantitative evaluation and maintenance, and (3) public justification were discussed and related to the attributes that characterize the educated person.

O'Neill, J. (1983). Examinations and quality control. In J. R. Warren (Ed.), *Meeting the new demand for standards* (pp. 69–79). San Francisco, CA: Jossey-Bass.

> The author identifies the current crisis in accreditation as the unwillingness or inability of higher education to define minimum standards. He

advocates the use of departmentally created comprehensive examinations or use of the GRE or other standardized tests to evaluate outcomes.

Osigweh, C. A. B. (1986). A value-added model of measuring performance. *College Teaching, 34*, 28–33.

> Article concerning Northeast Missouri State University's development of a way of knowing its effectiveness through a method of assessment that focuses on the value added to the student's knowledge and personality. Competence testing and attitudinal assessment are used. The effects on curriculum and instruction are outlined. A figure of the model used at NMSU and a table of midprogram assessment results using ACT Testing are provided.

Palola, E. G., & Lehmann, T. (1976). Improving student outcomes and institutional decision making with PERC. In O. T. Lenning (Ed.), *Improving educational outcomes.* San Francisco, CA: Jossey-Bass.

> For colleges and universities who take evaluation seriously and who want to build relationships between program effectiveness and related costs, the author indicates certain minimum tasks must be completed. Four tasks are briefly described.

Pascarella, E. T. (1980). Student faculty informal contact and college outcomes. *Review of Educational Research, 50*, 545–595.

> Provides a critical review and synthesis of research on the association between student-faculty informal nonclass contact and various outcomes of college academic performance, intellectual development, personal development, educational career aspirations, college satisfaction, and institutional integration. A table of sample independent variable, dependent variable, controls, and results for studies reviewed for this paper is provided.

Petersen, D. G. (1981). Process and outcomes. In I. M. Shimffer (Ed.), *Quality—Higher Education's Principal Challenge* (pp. 57–63). Washington, DC: American Council on Education.

> The author argues for continuing to improve the use of the process criterion while accelerating attempts at evaluation based on evidence of successful outcomes.

Rotem, A., Craig, P., Cox, K., & Ewan, C. (1981). In search of criteria for the assessment of medical education. *Medical Education, 15*, 85–91.

> This study was performed to assess whether an undergraduate educational curriculum is relevant. Subjects were individuals involved in medical

education or health science administration in Australia. They were asked to suggest five major criteria for judging whether a medical undergraduate program is relevant or not and to say whether they felt current curricula meet these criteria.

Schomberg, S. F., Hendel, D. D., & Bassett, C. L. (1983). Using the college outcomes measures project to measure college outcomes. *Alternative Higher Education, 7*(2), 95–104.

> Research report of the use of the College Outcome Measures Project (COMP) to compare graduates of traditional and nontraditional programs.

Stark, J. S., Lowther, M. A. (1986). *Executive summary of the University of Michigan professional preparation study project survey.* Ann Arbor, MI: University of Michigan, Center for the Study of Higher and Postsecondary Education.

> Summary report of ongoing research to improve understanding of diverse professional programs in colleges and universities. One of several objectives was to explore criteria for measuring student outcomes. Survey respondents—faculty from 10 professional fields including nursing—identified 11 potential outcomes for professional preparation and indicated professional competence was slightly more important than professional attitudes.

Stark, J. S., Lowther, M. A., & Hagerty, B. M. K. (1986). *Responsive professional education: Balancing outcomes and opportunities.* ASHE-ERIC Higher Education Report No. 3. Washington, DC: Association for the Study of Higher Education.

> One hundred twelve-page report that reviews the similarities and differences of the curricula of 12 professional fields. After reviewing over 300 publications, the authors divide their study into professional competencies and professional attitudes. In the analysis of six professional competencies and five attitudinal outcomes, the purpose and successes or failures of professional education are discussed along with the larger issues of evaluating competence and measuring outcomes for other curricula.

Terenzini, P. T., Theophilides, C., & Lorang, W. G. (1984). Influences on students' perceptions of their personal development during the first three years of college. *Research in Higher Education, 21*, 178–194.

> Longitudinal ex post facto study to (1) determine whether students' perceptions of their personal development are related to their college experiences after controlling for their pre-college characteristics, (2) determine whether the reported growth varies over three years of college, and (3) as-

sess whether the sources of influence on students' reported personal development vary from one year to another.

Troutt, W. E. (1981). Relationship between regional accrediting association standards and educational quality. In R. I. Miller (Ed.), *Institutional assessment for self improvement.* San Francisco, CA: Jossey-Bass.

> The author notes that regional accreditation standards never required explicit standards for students. He recommends the focus be upon student performance at graduation. In this way assessing institutional performance would be a matter of checking demonstrated student achievement against the descriptions of degrees awarded.

Turnbull, W. W. (1985, November/December). Are they learning anything in college? *Change,* 23, 26.

> Article emphasizes the need for assessment of higher education. The author encourages the development of assessment strategies that can be used by many institutions and emphasizes the need for measurement of performance at entry, and at the end of each academic year, and at graduation.

Young, K., & Chambers, C. (1980). *Accrediting agency approaches to academic program evaluation.* San Francisco, CA: Jossey-Bass.

> The authors emphasize the need for the development of statements of educational outcomes that are clear and precise and that lend themselves to evaluation. This does not necessarily mean measurement, because some of the most important outcomes of the teaching-learning process cannot easily be measured; however, they can be evaluated.